Tell Me What to Eat
If I Have
Diabetes

Third Edition

Tell Me What to Eat
If I Have
Diabetes

Third Edition

Nutrition You Can Live With

By Elaine Magee, MPH, RD

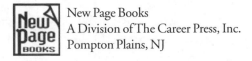

New Page Books
A Division of The Career Press, Inc.
Pompton Plains, NJ

TELL ME WHAT TO EAT IF I HAVE DIABETES
EDITED BY DIANA GHAZZAWI
TYPESET BY GINA TALUCCI
Cover design by Lu Rossman/Digi Dog Design NYC
Printed in the U.S.A.

To order this title, please call toll-free 1-800-CAREER-1 (NJ and Canada: 201-848-0310) to order using VISA or MasterCard, or for further information on books from Career Press.

The Career Press, Inc., 220 West Parkway, Unit 12
Pompton Plains, NJ 07444
www.careerpress.com
www.newpagebooks.com

Library of Congress Cataloging-in-Publication Data
Magee, Elaine.
    Tell me what to eat if I have diabetes : nutrition you can live with /
    by Elaine Magee. —3rd ed.
        p. cm.
    Includes index.
    ISBN 978-1-60163-021-6
    1. Non-insulin-dependent diabetes—Diet therapy. I. Title.

RC662.18.M34 2009
616.4'620654--dc22

                                                    2008032875

Contents

Introduction

If you've just been told you have diabetes, I hope you will find comfort in knowing that there has never been a better time than now to start managing and improving your diabetes. Researchers know more today than they did just five years ago about diet, insulin, other medications, complications, and more!

Let me tell you about what I call the "Diabetes Double Whammy" that comes from modern-day living. Insulin-resistant type 2 diabetes can be traced to the obesity epidemic that arose after World War II. The responsibility of making food for the family started shifting from the family kitchen to factories and restaurants, which tended to make high-fat, calorie-dense foods. On a large scale, people started consuming more calories on a daily basis at the same time that fewer calories were being burned in this modern-day technological age. The obvious solution to the Diabetes Double Whammy is moving food preparation back to the family kitchen as often as possible and staying physically active to increase the number of calories burned, in spite of living in this high-tech age.

Three known factors that increase the risk for type 2 diabetes are obesity, age, and lack of exercise. You can't do anything about age, but you can change the other two risk factors—obesity and exercise. In terms of dietary changes, the truth is that it would have been much easier to write this book if there were one specific diet to recommend for all persons with type 2 diabetes. But there isn't. All persons with type 2 diabetes are not created equal. Each person needs to work out his or her particular eating, exercise, or medication plan so that it translates into normal blood sugars in his or her particular body. Some people seem to have better blood sugars with meals low in fat, while others do better with meals richer in monounsaturated fat (in which 30 to 40 percent of calories come from fat). But no matter which type of person you are, you will still need the tools to make better meal choices and balance carbohydrates, fat, and fiber in your meal plan. I'll give you those tools. There are other food patterns and nutrients that seem to help most people with diabetes. I'll talk about those too.

Most diabetes specialists believe there are four keys to managing diabetes:

1. Monitoring your blood glucose levels.
2. Exercising regularly.
3. Wise meal planning.
4. Medication and prescriptions.

This book, *Tell Me What to Eat If I Have Diabetes, Third Edition*, will obviously spend the bulk of its pages on the third key. But don't be surprised if you find some tips on the first two as well. As a matter of fact, exercising regularly and monitoring your blood glucose are two of the 10 Food Steps to Freedom in Chapter 4.

I also wanted to introduce my latest book to you, *Food Synergy*, which is about how components within whole foods, and between different foods, work together in your body for maximum health benefits. For example, these are the possible foods or food partnerships with the type of synergy that might improve blood sugar control: fiber, whole grains, soluble fiber in oats, beans, and ground flaxseed. The following are foods with synergy that seems to help keep insulin levels steady: whole grains, soluble fiber in oats, soy protein, and ground flaxseed.

I hope, as you read *Tell Me What to Eat If I Have Diabetes, Third Edition,* you will feel as though I am holding your hand and walking with you as you begin this journey. I know how difficult, and sometimes depressing, having type 2 diabetes can be. I held my dad's hand through the last 20 years of having this disease. He wasn't very interested in helping his body live longer and better with diabetes. But, hopefully, you are. I wrote this book to help *you.*

The best gift I can give you is to help you feel great and get your diabetes under good control, all the while eating foods you love and enjoy. This book will get you closer to that goal. That is my promise.

Publisher's Note

This book is not intended as a substitute for medical advice. Readers are encouraged to consult with a doctor before following this or any other dietary advice.

Chapter 1

The Who, What, Where, Why, and How of Type 2 Diabetes

Diabetes is reaching epidemic proportions. It is the third or seventh leading cause of death in the United States, depending on whether you include the people with diabetes who die from related cardiovascular disease. Roughly 18 million Americans already have diabetes and many more will get it in the coming years as Baby Boomers age and the rise in adult and child obesity continues. Experts say that about eight to nine million Americans are totally unaware they even have diabetes. Often, they don't find out until fairly severe damage has been done to their bodies. What kind of damage? Uncontrolled diabetes is the leading cause of blindness, kidney failure, and leg amputations. But a wise diabetes educator once told me that "controlled" diabetes is the leading cause of…nothing! That's the truth and the good news.

Once you have diabetes, your risk for heart disease can be four times greater. So telling you what to eat for type 2 diabetes also has to include telling you what to eat to reduce your risk of heart disease. In fact, the types of food and meal choices that work best for diabetics (lower sugar, lower sodium, high fiber, lean meats and plant protein, fruits, and vegetables, with sources of monounsaturated fats and omega-3 fatty acids) are great for someone *without* diabetes who is just trying to eat right and prevent disease. The only difference is that someone *with* diabetes needs to carefully control and monitor his or her blood sugar and, therefore, sometimes needs to keep count of carbohydrate, fiber, and fat grams throughout his or her day.

Q: What is insulin, and what does it normally do in the body?

Insulin is a hormone normally produced as needed by the pancreas, and one of its major jobs is helping get glucose (energy) into various body cells. When blood glucose levels rise, the pancreas makes more insulin and releases it into the bloodstream. The insulin then causes body cells to remove the excess glucose that is circulating in the blood. In the liver and skeletal muscle cells, the insulin encourages the production of glycogen (the storage form of glucose). In the liver and fat cells, insulin encourages fat production (stored energy). At the same time, insulin discourages the breakdown of body fat for energy (lipolysis), causing the body to rely more heavily on the recently ingested carbohydrates for current energy needs.

Q: What is type 2 diabetes?

Type 2 diabetes is a metabolic disorder resulting from the body's inability to make enough or properly use insulin. As discussed, insulin is a hormone that triggers body cells to convert sugar, starches, and other foods into energy. Type 2 diabetes is a result of insulin resistance and can occur when the body produces plenty of insulin, but the insulin cannot do its job. For some reason, the cells in the body have become resistant to insulin. In most cases, being overweight or obese for a period of time could bring on the insulin resistance, but there are people who are obese for many years who never develop diabetes. So scientists suspect that some people have a genetic predisposition, that their particular genes make them more likely to develop type 2 diabetes under certain conditions, such as with aging, weight gain, or an inactive lifestyle. About 90 to 95 percent of people with diabetes have type 2.

Q: What are the warning signs of type 2 diabetes?

Some people with type 2 don't have obvious signs, but they could have any of the following symptoms:

- Frequent infections.
- Blurred vision.
- Cuts that are slow to heal.
- Tingling and/or numbness in hands or feet.
- Unusual thirst.
- Frequent urination.
- Extreme hunger.
- Unusual weight loss.
- Extreme fatigue.
- Irritability.

Q: Why do some people get type 2 diabetes?

Insulin resistance is the common cause, but not all people with type 2 diabetes are created equal. Most people with type 2 diabetes start with the potential to develop the disease, such as a genetic predisposition based on family history or ethnicity, that eventually becomes manifested through environmental factors such as aging, weight gain, or a sedentary lifestyle, all leading to insulin resistance.

Q: Can changing my lifestyle improve my type 2 diabetes?

In the past five to 10 years, important studies have been published documenting how good exercise is for people with diabetes or who are at risk for developing it. Well, recently the National Institute for Health did a study to find out whether the onset of diabetes in a high-risk group could actually be prevented. They compared a lifestyle modification program that included healthy changes, such as nutrition, exercise and a minimal amount of weight loss (Hello! This is the Elaine Magee way of living!) with a treatment program that relied on medication. Guess what happened? The lifestyle program ended up trumping the treatment program! The lifestyle program was twice as good, twice as powerful, with an almost 60 percent reduction in the onset of diabetes, compared with those using medications, which reduced it by 30 percent.

All in favor of working out today and enjoying a nice high-fiber dinner with smart fats featured say aye!

Q: Is type 2 diabetes an outcome of nurture or nature?

Behavior, rather than genetics, may provide the key to reducing a woman's risk of developing type 2 diabetes. Results from the Nurses' Health Study suggest that the majority—an estimated nine out of 10 cases—of type 2 diabetes could be prevented by weight loss, regular physical activity, healthy diet, abstinence from smoking, and moderate consumption of alcohol (half to one drink per day for women). The risk reduction was similar for women with and without a family history of the disease. Because diabetes is a major risk factor for cardiovascular disease, such modifications may help prevent heart disease. Researchers following nearly 85,000 nurses for 16 years concluded that an estimated 91 percent of the 3,300 new cases of type 2 diabetes diagnosed during the study could have been prevented by lifestyle modifications.

Excess body fat was the single most important risk factor in the development of type 2 diabetes. The heavier a woman was, the greater her risk of developing the disease, even if she was at the high end of a normal BMI (body mass index, a measure of body fat). An estimated 97 million Americans are overweight or obese, making them all at an increased risk for diabetes.

Lack of physical activity was also a significant risk factor, independent of body weight. Conversely, women who exercised seven or more hours weekly cut their risk by 50 percent, compared with sedentary women. About 75 percent of the U.S. population is considered to be minimally engaged in physical activity or daily exercise.

The women at lowest risk ate a diet high in cereal fiber and polyunsaturated fats, and low in saturated and trans fat. They abstained from smoking and drank moderately [Nurses' Health Study 9 (2002)].

Q: What are the end-points of uncontrolled diabetes?

Uncontrolled diabetes is the leading cause of blindness in working-age adults in the United States, accounting for 24,000 new blind persons every year. The National Eye Institute estimates that 90 percent of lost vision is preventable. Uncontrolled diabetes is the leading cause of end-stage renal disease in the United States. Approximately 28,000 patients with diabetes develop end-stage renal disease every year. With all the current therapies now available, future cases of end-stage renal disease are probably preventable. Uncontrolled diabetes is the leading cause of non-traumatic lower extremity amputations in the United States. Keep in mind that about 95 percent are thought to be preventable, another incentive to manage your diabetes well!

Q: How will this book help?

I know it takes some time to really accept that you now have diabetes. This may take a few months or a few years, depending on the person. A good friend of mine was in what you could call "diabetic denial" for about two years—not exercising, not really paying attention to her blood glucose or what she ate. She was one of the first people to whom I gave a copy of the first edition of this book. Every time I would see her, I would ask if she had read it. She would always have an excuse.

Finally one day she said, "I guess I better start acting like a diabetic." Almost overnight she started monitoring her blood glucose; counting carbohydrates, fat, and fiber; and working some exercise into her busy workweek. She feels much better now. Guess what? She had finally read the book.

If you are reading this book right now, chances are you have accepted that diabetes is now a part of your life. You want to make it work for you. You want to manage your blood glucose, reduce your risk of heart disease, and just plain feel better. Because you *want* to make changes, this book can help.

Q: How do I get my type 2 diabetes under control?

Many diabetes specialists believe there are four keys to diabetes management success:

1. Monitoring blood glucose levels.

You need to monitor your blood glucose, because that's how you know right away if you are keeping your blood glucose near normal. And you need to keep your blood glucose near normal if you want to protect your body from developing diabetic complications further down the line. If your healthcare team knows how your blood sugar is being affected from day to day, they can help fine-tune your medications, your eating plan, and your exercise routine.

Measuring your blood glucose will tell you rather quickly whether your treatments (diet, exercise, and pharmacological) are working for you. Make sure someone on your healthcare team clearly demonstrates how to measure your glucose and how to record it so it can be referred to easily at follow-up visits.

This is very important to the management of diabetes. Next to the discovery of insulin, the ability to monitor blood sugars was the biggest breakthrough in the treatment of diabetes.

The American Diabetes Association recommends a goal of 90 to 130 milligrams per deciliter (mg/dL) for preprandial (pre-meal) blood glucose levels in adults with diabetes. The American Association of Clinical Endocrinologists recommends that adults aim for a preprandial blood glucose goal of less than or equal to 110 mg/dL.

Generally blood glucose levels are taken two hours after a meal, which is thought to be when the blood glucose concentrations are at their peak. The American Diabetes Association recommends less than 180 mg/dL for peak postprandial (post-meal) glucose levels. The American Association of Clinical Endocrinologists recommends adults aim for a postprandial goal of less than or equal to 140 mg/dL.

Hemoglobin A1c levels are directly related to blood glucose concentrations over the previous two to three months. The A1c test is often given twice each year in stable patients and four or more times a year in patients where glycemic control is more challenging. The A1c test goal is less than or equal to 7 percent. The following table shows the mean blood glucose levels that correlate with various hemoglobin A1c test results:

Hemoglobin A1c	Mean Blood Glucose
6 percent	135 mg/dL
7 percent	170 mg/dL
8 percent	205 mg/dL
9 percent	240 mg/dL
10 percent	275 mg/dL

2. Exercising regularly.

Exercise can actually help control blood glucose levels. Exercise depresses insulin production and also prompts skeletal muscle cells to take in more glucose from the bloodstream. With more glucose in your muscle cells, you can produce more energy so that your muscles can continue to work.

Besides helping to control blood glucose levels, exercise improves the cardiovascular system, thus reducing the risk of heart disease, and also encourages weight loss, which can have big benefits for people with diabetes.

3. Planning your meals wisely.

This is the key that this book will give you the most help with. It will help you follow a plan that keeps your personal blood glucose levels normal, protects against heart disease and weight gain, and doesn't make you feel deprived. This book, though, is not about telling you the one and only way to eat; no one diet is best for all people with diabetes. Every person has different risk factors (obesity, hypertension, high triglycerides, kidney dialysis, etc.) that need to be considered. I will tell you generally which foods or meals will be more likely to cause higher blood sugars. But when it comes right down to it, every person is affected by the same food or meal a little differently. Chalk it up to unexplained individual differences.

Generally, many people with diabetes seem to tolerate a more moderate-carbohydrate (around 45 percent of calories from carbohydrate), moderate-fat (around 35 percent of calories from fat) way of eating. Of course, this eating plan requires using mostly canola oil, olive oil, and avocado, which are high in more desirable monounsaturated fats. Having a couple servings of fish, which is rich in omega-3 fatty acids, each week wouldn't hurt either.

4. Work with your doctor and dietitian on medications and prescriptions specific to your medical condition.

It's important to work with your healthcare team particularly if insulin is part of your treatment plan.

Is there such a thing as too much insulin when it comes to managing or treating type 2 diabetes? Some researchers believe that giving more insulin can lead to increased body fat, as they discussed in a March 2008 press release at UT Southwestern Medical Center. While high doses of insulin may lower glucose levels, it will also increase the fatty molecules and may cause organ damage, according to new research. Dr. Roger Unger, professor of Internal Medicine at UT Southwestern Medical Center, now believes, after investigating diabetes, obesity, and insulin resistance for more than 50 years, that intensive insulin therapy may not be best for obese patients with insulin-resistant type 2 diabetes, because it increases the fatty acids that cause diabetes. The most rational therapy, he suggests, eliminates excess calories, thereby reducing the amount of insulin in the blood and the synthesis of the fatty acids stimulated by the high insulin levels.

According to Unger, one treatment option to be considered before giving insulin is bariatric surgery. For many with type 2 diabetes, the excess body fat is causing insulin resistance and killing the insulin-producing beta cells in the pancreas. The aim, then, might be to correct the insulin resistance by reducing body fat. So it's quite possible that for overweight patients with poorly controlled, insulin-resistant type 2 diabetes, weight loss and major lifestyle changes may actually be more effective than intensive insulin therapy.

But this remains a hot issue among diabetes researchers, so stay tuned because Chinese researchers recently reported that when intensive insulin therapy was given to people just diagnosed with type 2 diabetes, it seemed to improve B-cell (the cells in the pancreas that produce insulin) function compared to using oral hypoglycemic agents.

Q: Where can I go for more information?

To find a Certified Diabetes Educator (CDE) in your area (many provide individual consultations and some offer classes for diabetics), go to *www.diabeteseducator.org*.

For a list of registered dietitians with expertise in diabetes (RD, CDE) in your area, contact the American Dietetic Association's National Center for Nutrition and Dietetics at 800-366-1655 or visit its Website *www.eatright.org*.

The American Diabetes Association maintains a hotline at 800-DIABETES (800-342-2383), and information on types of diabetes is available by mail and fax, and fromstaff members. The association's Website is *www.diabetes.org*.

Hopefully your local diabetes center or clinic has a referral sheet available, filled with local numbers for everything from diabetes support groups and counselors to dietitians, diabetes educators, fitness clubs, and personal trainers. If they don't, find somewhere that does. Many hospitals have diabetes support groups, and that is a great starting place.

Chapter 2

Top 3 Profiles of Type 2 Diabetes

I know you may feel as if you have been wearing the label "type 2 diabetes" lately and that health professionals and other people like to lump all type 2s together. The truth is that people with type 2 diabetes come in different shapes and sizes and with different health risks and medical problems. Your health risks and medical problems, in addition to having type 2 diabetes, also define what needs to be done food-wise to help you feel better and live longer. It is important we get these other issues on the table so that you can get a better idea of what your personal diet and food priorities are and how your type 2 diabetes might differ from that of others.

There are certain profiles that stand out in people with type 2 diabetes. I will discuss a few in this chapter.

1. Waiting to lose weight

The good news is that losing weight greatly decreases your risk for type 2 diabetes and can help bring your blood sugar under control if you already have type 2. The challenging part is actually losing the weight and then keeping it off. Let me first say, you are not alone. I have spent most of my adult life waiting to lose weight.

I understand how difficult it is. I know that often thin people actually eat more and exercise less than thicker people (but who's counting?). I know what it is like to eat healthy, exercise every day, and still not lose weight.

I know the majority of Americans are considered "overweight." But what shocked me was that survey data by the National Center for Health Statistics in 1988–1991 showed a dramatic increase of about eight pounds in mean body weight of U.S. adults since the last survey was conducted (1976–1980). It didn't matter which gender, age, or cultural group you looked at—weight gain still followed.

How can this be? Atkins, Jenny Craig, Weight Watchers, Slim Fast, and other billion-dollar dieting giants have been waging war against weight gain for decades now! Never before have more reduced-fat foods been available. Getting back to the basics of weight control sheds some light on this rather sore subject.

As you've probably heard, one of the first questions related to weight control asks whether the "calories in" equal the "calories out." That's because the net effect of excess calories (more than our current body needs), even in the form of protein, is going to increase the amount of fat put into storage (body fat). We know that most Americans haven't exactly been increasing their "calories out" side of the equation. Due to a combination of modern-life factors (television, long commutes, computers, etc.), Americans have become more sedentary.

What about the "calories in" portion? True, the average person ate less fat as a percentage of total calories during the survey period (down from 36 to 34 percent), but the amount of total daily calories went up an average of 231 calories compared to 1976–1980. Aaah, now we're getting to the real million-dollar question: Why would Americans suddenly increase their total daily calories at a time when the country has never been more obsessed with dieting and more concerned about healthy eating?

Maybe because a large chunk of the American population is actively dieting at any one time, they continue to ride the unfortunate weight roller coaster of strict dieting and obsession—deprivation, bingeing and guilt, strict dieting and obsession—over and over again. Studies show that when people diet, the vast majority of them eventually gain the weight back—and then some. Maybe some of these eight pounds are the "and then some" from a country that chronically diets.

So what are we going to do about it?

- **Stop dieting!** We know it doesn't work. We know it actually works against you.

- **Eat when you are hungry and stop when you are comfortable.** When we "diet" we force ourselves *not* to listen to our natural hunger cues. When we do this, we also tend *not* to listen to our "comfortable" cues. We react to deprivation and not listening to hunger by overeating at times. In order to stop overeating, we need to stop dieting and start listening to when our body truly is hungry and truly is comfortable. But, unfortunately, all of this may be a little trickier for people with type 2 diabetes. The biochemistry of the disease is thought to alter natural hunger regulation, so you may have to pay attention to hunger and eating until you are comfortable within the specific plan that you have worked out with your Certified Diabetes Educator to keep your blood sugars normal.

- **Beware of calories you are drinking.** Your body tends not to feel satisfied by liquid calories, and opting for healthier beverages is an easy way to trim excess calories.

- **Slow down; you're eating too fast.** It takes at least 20 minutes for your brain to get the message that your stomach is officially "comfortable" and that you should stop eating. If you eat slowly, the brain has a chance to catch up with the stomach and you are more likely not to overeat. Here are some tips to help slow you down during your meal:

  - Slow down your meal and chew slowly too.

  - Don't eat standing up, your brain and stomach are more likely to register that you are eating if you are relaxed and enjoying the meal.

  - Drink a 12-ounce glass of water before eating a meal.

- **Start exercising!** Exercising helps your body in so many ways. It is one of the fastest ways to increase your "calories out" side of the equation. (See Step #10 in Chapter 4 for information about how to exercise if you don't like to exercise.)

- **Start counting** carbohydrates, fats, and fiber as often as you can to gain close control of your blood sugars. I know counting is a big pain. But you don't have to do it all the time for the rest of your life. You might start counting your carbohydrates, fat, and fiber every day until your blood sugars are under control. Then you can do "check in" counting—about every week or every month if your blood sugars are staying within normal limits.

Logging in what you eat and your exercise will also help you and your dietitian or Certified Diabetes Educator better understand what small changes might take place to encourage weight loss.

To diet or not to diet

When the holidays have finally passed, 'tis the season to get dieting. It's the American way. But when it comes to shopping for a "diet," it's buyer beware, according to a report from the Federal Trade Commission, released September 17, 2002. The researchers found that 55 percent of the weight-loss advertisements made at least one false or unsubstantiated claim. Does this really surprise us? Nearly half the ads claimed you could lose weight without dieting and exercise.

All fad diets promoting fast and furious weight loss generally don't work over the long haul. Some of us have already figured this out on our own but we can't quite stop ourselves from perking up and asking "How'd you do it?" every time we hear someone say they lost 20 pounds. We can't quite tune out the countless TV commercials we see daily for weight-loss programs and products.

If you are going to partake of a fad diet in the new year, go in forewarned that with fad diets, weight loss is temporary. A USDA study found that pretty much any fad diet will help you take off the pounds, but there's not much evidence that they'll help you keep the weight off. Fad diets often work in the short run, because they are low-calorie diets in disguise.

Weight loss fact: The only way to lose weight without medication or surgery is to consume less energy (calories) than your body needs. No magic ingredients or food combinations will change this basic metabolic fact.

But most people who successfully lose weight return to their old eating habits sooner or later and regain most of the lost weight within two years (Denke M. "Metabolic effects of high-protein, low-carbohydrate diets" *Am J Cardiol* [2001];88:59–61). That's why the way of eating you choose needs to be practical and healthful for a lifetime. Most fad diets are not.

Nobody wants to hear this but, there is no miracle remedy or diet for losing weight. Your best bet is to stick with the proven method of eating less, eating healthier, and exercising more.

So say you are ready to try to eat less, eat healthy, and exercise more. Which "diet" or way of eating is the best way to do that? The popular low-carbohydrate/high-protein way? The low-fat/ higher-carbohydrate way? Or, the moderate fat way (but emphasizing the better fat, carbohydrate, and protein choices)? Each will work in the short run as long as the calories you take in are less than the calories you are expending. But, healthwise, which is best?

Q: Where are the fruits and vegetables?

Instead of "Where's the beef?" one crucial question to ask when looking at these different diets is "Where are the fruits and vegetables?" Recent studies have shown that the obesity levels are lowest among those who eat seven or more servings of fruits and vegetables a day (key finding from new research from the Produce for Better Health Foundation, Press Release October 21, 2002). And perhaps it isn't a coincidence that as Americans have been getting fatter over the last 10 years, fruit and vegetable consumption has declined nearly 14 percent, nationwide, during the same period. We all know fruits and vegetables are good for us. Well, guess what: they are mostly carbohydrate (vegetables will have some plant protein too).

A cup of steamed broccoli contains 44 calories, 4.5 grams protein, 8 grams carbohydrate, .5 grams of fat, and 4.7 grams of fiber. And a large apple contains 125 calories, .4 grams protein, 32 grams carbohydrate, .7 grams of fat, and 4.2 grams fiber. Both are brimming with a good dose of healthful carbohydrate, complete with fiber.

Q: Are you losing fat, lean body mass, or body water?

No one will argue that the main goal of weight loss is to lose body fat and not lean body mass (muscle). Water loss is fast and temporary, so eventually your body is going to need to restore the balance of water and will gain lost water pounds back.

The ideal weight-loss diet should provide enough carbohydrate to prevent protein/muscle breakdown, enough good-quality protein to meet the normal needs of protein turnover, and enough fat to meet essential fatty acid requirements.

The following covers each of these three major "diet" groups, their strengths and their weaknesses, and some tips for you to keep in mind should you decide (after consulting your doctor or dietitian) that's the program for you.

High protein/low carbohydrate. Atkins, South Beach, The Zone, Protein Power, Sugar Busters—do these diets sound familiar? These types of diets do encourage fast weight loss in the first week. Though what's initially happening here is mostly water loss. The body needs a constant supply of glucose energy, so without a lot of carbohydrates in the diet, body glycogen stores (the way the body stores some extra carbohydrates) are used up. For each gram of glycogen lost, two to four grams of body water is lost as well. One recent study demonstrated that the greater weight loss on a low-carbohydrate/high-protein diet plan is accounted for by losses in body water (Denke M. "Metabolic effects of high-protein, low-carbohydrate diets." *Am J Cardiol* [2001]; 88:59–61).

The American Heart Association has officially cautioned the public on high-protein diets. In an advisory to clinicians, it concluded that people who follow high-protein diets are at risk for "compromised vitamin and mineral intake, as well as potential cardiac, renal, bone, and liver abnormalities overall" (Circulation, 104, no. 15, (2001);1869–74). According to this American Heart Association Science Advisory report, "the beneficial effects on blood lipids and insulin resistance are due to the weight loss, not the change in caloric composition." The advisory also reminds us that there are no long-term scientific studies to support the overall efficacy and safety of the various and sundry high-protein diets.

One *plus* with this type of diet is that you can lose weight fast, which can give some people the impetus they need to make longer-term changes in their eating habits and lifestyle. But losing weight too fast can be a problem too. When weight loss is too fast, changes in body composition, especially the loss of lean body mass, can compound the problem of being overweight in the long run. When you lose weight fast, you tend to lose some lean body mass (muscle protein), but when you gain the weight back fast, it tends to come back as mostly body fat.

The other plus: there is some evidence that higher-protein diets are more satiating. People feel fuller and tend to eat less after a meal with a high-protein content (more than 25 percent calories from protein). High-protein foods tend to move more slowly from the stomach to the intestine than high-carbohydrate (refined) foods, so your stomach tends to feel full longer.

According to one report, two of the five high-protein diets on the market score slightly better nutritionally than the others. The Zone and Sugar Busters diets at least do not severely restrict carbohydrate to less than 100 grams a day and total fat and saturated fat are not excessive (greater than 30 percent calories from fat and 10 percent calories from saturated fat). (Circulation, 2001, Vol. 104, No. 15, pp 1869–74.)

The bottom line: this way of eating *can't* and *shouldn't* be continued over a long period of time. These diets are generally associated with higher intakes of fat, saturated fat, and cholesterol, if the protein choices come mostly from animal sources. In the long term, very-high-protein diets may increase the risk of atherosclerosis (one study showed that this diet increases serum cholesterol levels and may increase the risk of coronary heart disease by more than 50 percent with long-term use (*J Am Coll Nutr* [2000]; 19:578–590). Dr. Thomas Lee, MD, commented in the March 2002 issue of the "Harvard Heart Letter" that for most people eating a high-protein diet (including lots of cheese, red meat, and other high-fat foods), their cholesterol levels, especially LDL (bad) cholesterol, go way up and that limiting foods that lower LDLs (such as high-fiber plant foods) only intensifies this problem.

Here's another fact that you need to keep in mind with high-protein diets: the more protein you eat, the more calcium you excrete. High-protein diets, when followed for a long time, can increase your risk of osteoporosis by increasing calcium excretion, and place an extra stress on the kidneys, which are removing high amounts of nitrogen waste products from the high-protein intake, particularly during times of high water loss from perspiration or low fluid intake contributing to dehydration.

Short-term consequences of following a diet that encourages high protein and fatty foods include dehydration, diarrhea, weakness, headaches, dizziness, and bad breath. This type of diet also tends not to include sufficient fruits and vegetables for overall good health.

Where does the South Beach Diet fit into this? Similar to the Atkins Diet, the South Beach Diet is low in carbohydrates during its "Phase 1." But in the second phase, the plan legalizes healthful carbohydrates such as whole grains, high-fiber cereal, and most fruit, and allows sparing amounts of chocolate, red wine, and previously banished foods, such as low-fat yogurt.

High carbohydrate/very low fat. The biggest positive to this type of diet is that it can lead to healthy eating as long as the diet recommends high-fiber intakes, lower-glycemic-index carbohydrates (fruits, vegetables, beans, and whole grains tend to have lower glycemic indexes), and provides sufficient essential fatty acids and fat-soluble vitamins from the fats that are eaten.

Another plus is that the diet quality tends to be better with this type of diet compared to the low-carbohydrate diets. A U.S. study of popular diets demonstrated that the diet quality (measured by dietary variety and intake of five food groups, fat, saturated fat, and sodium) is higher in high-carbohydrate diets and lowest in low-carbohydrate diets. The same study also detected another plus to high-carbohydrate eating: body mass index (BMI) is lower in people following high-carbohydrate diets and highest in people on low-carbohydrate diets (Kennedy et al., "Popular diets: correlation to health, nutrition, and obesity" *JADA* 101 [2001]: 411–420).

The trouble with a high-carbohydrate/low-fat diet is that some might be tempted to fill up on higher-glycemic-index carbohydrates (refined starchy foods and concentrated sugar), which are rapidly digested and can cause a large increase in blood glucose and insulin after meals. Some clinical trials have reported less weight loss on high-glycemic-index diets compared to low-glycemic-index diets and some short-term feeding studies found that as glycemic index goes down, satiety (a satisfied feeling of fullness) tends to go up. (Pawlak et al., "Should obese patients be counseled to follow a low-glycemic-index diet?" *Obes Rev* 3, no. 4 [2002]: 235–43)

The bottom line: choose mostly smart carbohydrates (higher fiber, higher nutrient carbohydrates with lower glycemic indexes) and make sure you are getting enough protein and fat (olive oil, canola oil, fish, etc.) to meet your body's needs.

A moderate, more balanced way of eating. This way of eating tends not to be studied as a "diet," so there is very little research on this type of diet and weight loss. But if you combined the best part of the high-carbohydrate diet with the best part of the high-protein diet would you have the best of both worlds? In one recent study, a low-fat diet with 25 percent calories from protein was found to produce a significant reduced calorie intake and greater weight and fat loss over a six-month period compared to a low-fat diet with a lower-protein intake—12 percent calories from protein (*Int J Obes Relat Metab Disord* 23 [1999]: 528–536). That sounds encouraging.

If this way of eating emphasizes the higher fiber, nutrient-rich carbohydrate foods (whole grains, beans, fruits, and vegetables) and the lower-fat protein sources (lean meats, fish, skinless poultry, low-fat dairy, and/or vegetable protein sources such as beans, whole grains, nuts, and seeds) and uses some of the more favorable cooking fats (olive oil and canola oil), this diet is clearly the best of both "diet" worlds.

Look for the following in a weight-loss diet:

- Does it consider your current habits, preferences, and risk factors?

- Does it set realistic weight-loss goals (one to two pounds per week)?

- Does it have a daily intake of *at least 45 percent calories from carbohydrate?* For a woman eating at least 1,200 calories this would compute to at least 135 grams of carbohydrate a day, and 169 grams for a man eating at least 1,500 calories.

- Does it have a carbohydrate intake of *at least* 150 grams per day?

- Does it include all of the food groups?

- Does it emphasize fiber?

- Does it recommend regular exercise?

- Is it based on changing lifelong eating habits?

2. I have couch potato-itis

If the first thing doctors told you to do after being diagnosed with type 2 diabetes was "lose weight," then the second thing they probably told you was to "start exercising." The bottom line is that physical activity can make the difference between losing weight and not losing weight, blood sugar control and out-of-control blood sugars, going on insulin and not having to go on insulin, taking a high dose of insulin and taking a lower dose of insulin. Regular exercise has been shown to lower high triglycerides levels in the blood and lower high blood pressure after only 10 weeks. The risk of heart attack and cancer also decreases with regular exercise.

Exercise does much more than reduce risk factors; it has psychological benefits, too. It just plain makes you feel better. It tends to encourage better sleep, and it gives you more energy throughout the day. It helps you feel better about your body, even if pounds haven't been lost, and it helps reduce depression and stress.

I can go over and over all the various and sundry benefits (immediate and down-the-road) of exercise and physical activity, and I can even hold your hand and follow you around for a month helping you get in the habit of exercising. But sooner or later it is all going to come back to one person: you. Ultimately, you have to take responsibility for yourself.

The first step, other than accepting that you have diabetes, is to commit to trying exercise for one month, remembering to start slowly. To see major benefits in your blood sugar control, exercising five to six times a week (even if it is just for 15 minutes each time) is helpful. At the end of one month you should hopefully have experienced many of the psychological and physiological benefits to exercise and you will be, let's hope, adequately "hooked." So let's look at how to get started:

- Visit your doctor and make sure you can proceed with your plans to start exercising.

- Don't make it a big weight-loss contest—focus on health and gaining better control of your blood sugar.

- It has to be fun or you are definitely not going to stick with it.

- Find out what your exercise preferences/needs are and try to consider them when making your exercise plans.

- Do you like exercising outdoors or indoors?

- Do you like to exercise alone, with a partner, or with a group?

- Do you like the gym atmosphere?

- What time of day would you be most likely to stick to exercising?

- Do you have any physical limitations that need to be considered? If you have joint limitations, for example, water aerobics or swimming can be a great starting place.

- What do you like to do? Even if your answer is watching television or talking, they can be worked into your exercise program. If you like to talk, walking with a partner might be the ticket. It you like to watch television, then home exercise equipment that you can do in the comfort of your family room or bedroom might be your most practical option.

Every little bit helps

Even if you can't imagine exercising 30 minutes or more in one sitting, split it up into three 10-minute mini-workouts. Ten minutes of activity here and there does add up to health benefits for your body. Any way that you can increase your activity throughout your day will help your cause.

Here are some tips to keep you exercising month after month:

- Wherever you choose to exercise (gym, park, or pool) it should be **no more than 20 minutes away** from your home or work.

- **Start an exercise journal** or incorporate the information into your "A Day at a Glance" chart on pages 88–90. You will be able to see progress. You will also be able to trace back situations when the exercise helped lower your blood sugars.

- **Have a plan B.** Have some indoor options for exercise planned. During the winter, it might be too cold to exercise outdoors, or it might get dark earlier and you are concerned about safety. Or perhaps you get stuck in traffic and don't get home in time to make your exercise class. Your plan B could be riding your stationary bike or playing one of your exercise videos.

- **Plan variety** into your exercise schedule. If you go to a dance class two times a week, you might want to add a walking workout a couple times a week. I have three different types of exercise I do in any week (what can I say, I get bored easily). I go to Jazzercise two to three times a week and fill the rest of my week in with walks around the neighborhood and evening rides on my stationary bike (while I watch my favorite nighttime television shows).

- **Make different types of activity part of your normal day.** These may include walking the dog, walking to the mailbox, taking a flight of stairs, or walking during part of your lunch break.

- **Check in with a personal trainer every three months.** They can give you specific things you can do, given your personal experiences and preferences. A "check in" session will run you about $30 to $100, and you can call the American College of Sports Medicine for a list of personal trainers in your area (*www.acsm.org*).

- To keep yourself from getting bored, don't be afraid to **try something new**. You could sign up for a class with your local parks and recreation program or through a community college. You could try a session of country western dance class and then try yoga, water aerobics, tai chi, or tap the next session.

- You've got to **choose exercise that you actually enjoy**. Of course it is a matter of personal preference, but a large majority of people enjoy walking the most. It's easy, free, and only requires a pair of comfortable shoes. Look around your home or work for lakes or parks that you can walk around after dinner, during the lunch hour, or on the weekends.

- If you are the type of person who is inspired by reaching a goal each day, consider wearing a pedometer! Throughout the day you will see the numbers on your pedometer increase and if you have a certain number of steps to reach each day, this will really motivate many people to keep moving and walking! Talk to your doctor, but 10,000 steps is the total many very active people have at the end of the day after really trying hard to get those steps in. Your doctor might encourage you to start with 5,000 steps and work your way up to 10,000.

Home exercise equipment

Stationary and recumbent (in which your back is supported) bicycles are very successful with former couch potatoes. You can literally go from the couch to the bicycle. Position a fan in front of the bicycle if you like. There are a few things to consider when picking out an exercise bike:

- Make sure the seat is adjusted to your body correctly.

- Make sure the seat is wide and comfortable.

- If you opt for a stationary bike, consider the type where the fly wheel gives you a breeze (helping you to cool off) and the handles move (because this prevents leaning).

- Many people make the mistake of buying the inexpensive exercise equipment. I know this is tempting. To get the well-made equipment, the kind that will last a lifetime, it will run you around $800 (give or take a couple hundred). This is shocking, I know. But if you buy the cheaper stuff that creaks when you use it, it will inevitably break or you will tire of it quickly because it isn't as comfortable to use. Isn't buying one of the well-made pieces of equipment better than buying three cheaper pieces that you will stop using after a few months? Many stores offer payment plans in which the cost is about $20 to $30 a month. There are also places that sell used exercise equipment, which would shave quite a bit off the price.

Another home exercise no-no: don't buy exercise equipment through catalogs or television commercials. You want to try it out before you buy it. Literally get your sweats on and go to the sports equipment store. Tell them you want to try it out for 20 or 30 minutes. Only then will you be able to tell whether you can comfortably exercise on it for at least 30 minutes at home.

If you want to research the better designed pieces of exercise equipment, look up *Consumer Reports* at your local library—they rate exercise equipment every year. But remember the only way to know for sure how you like it is to just get on and try it.

3. The junk food junkie

Are you a junk food junkie? For food to qualify as "junk food" it usually contributes a high amount of calories for a low amount of nutritional value.

The problem with these types of foods (lots of calories within a small food volume, low fiber and water content, and low nutrients) is that they tend to cause a decrease in satiety (fullness and satisfaction when eating), which can encourage people to over consume calories, potentially leading to obesity. Sound familiar, America?

A big portion of what I would call "junk food" essentially falls into the categories of "snack food" and "fast food." Popular snack foods are usually either packaged or commercially prepared such as chips, cheese puffs, candy bars, snack cakes, and cookies. The contribution of snack-type food to our total calories consumes should not be underestimated. Between 1977 and 1996, the contribution of snack calories to total calories for American children between 2 and 5 years of age increased by 30 percent, according to an article in the Chile medical journal, *Revista Medica de Chile*. Junk food is also quickly purchased at fast-food chains across the country in the form of French fries, chicken nuggets, shakes, soda, etc., and we all know how pervasive fast food is in our current American culture. Then there are certain food categories such as breakfast cereals that seem innocent enough but include various products that could definitely be considered "junk food," being that they mostly contain sugar or high fructose corn syrup and white flour or milled corn.

Keep in mind that what is or is not considered "junk food" can depend on who you ask. Some might say pizza is junk food, for example, where as I personally don't consider it 100 percent junk food, because it contributes nutrients through real foods such as cheese and tomato sauce. Add whole-wheat or part whole-wheat pizza crust and some veggies as the topping and pizza completely exits the junk food category. You just can't compare the nutrients in pizza to the nutrients (or lack thereof) in a can of soda or a bag of chips.

Real food versus junk food

As if consuming the "junk" in junk food weren't bad enough, one of the worst health detriments of eating junk food is that it tends to replace real food—food that contributes necessary and beneficial nutrients. Got milk? When people drink lots of soda, for example, they are usually not getting plenty of low-fat dairy in their diets, along with other healthful beverages such as green tea or orange juice. When they are snacking on chips and cookies, they are usually not loading up on fruits and vegetables.

Taking the "junk" out of junk food

Opt for food and beverage choices, no matter where you are, that are comprised mostly of whole foods or ingredients that offer nutrients along with calories. Enjoy freshly squeezed orange juice or a whole-wheat bagel instead of soda or donuts. Buy a bean burrito, pizza topped with vegetables, or a grilled chicken sandwich on a whole grain bun instead of tortilla chips with processed cheese sauce, frozen pizza rolls, or fried chicken pieces and French fries. Choose a 100 percent whole-wheat cracker made with canola oil, for example, or make a cheese and fruit plate to snack on instead of a bowl of cheese puffs.

No matter what we do, typical fast food seems to make us eat more

Eating large amounts of food at a rapid rate is defined as "gorging" and this is NOT a healthy way to eat, in part because we are more likely to take in excessive amounts of calories. You want to eat in a slow and mindful way so food is enjoyed and your brain is aware of the eating process and is given time to tell your stomach when it is comfortable and satisfied. No good can come from eating large amounts of food fast, and this is exactly what people tend to do when they eat "fast food."

But is it the actual fast food that causes us to eat more than is needed or is it how much we are given and how we tend to eat fast food that seems to encourage gorging? A new study from the Children's Hospital in Boston used teens age 13 to 17 years and exposed them to three types of fast food meals (all including chicken nuggets, French fries, and cola). In one meal, they were served a lot of fast food at one time. In another, a lot of fast food was served in smaller portions, but almost at the same time. And in the third test meal, a lot of fast food was served in smaller portions over 15-minute intervals. The researchers analyzed how many calories were consumed by the teens in these three situations.

What they found was it didn't seem to matter how the large amount of fast food was served—the teens still ate about half of their daily calorie needs in that one meal. The researchers suggested that certain factors inherent to fast food might be promoting excessive calorie intake; for example, fast food is:

- Low in fiber
- High in palatability (pleasant tasting)
- High in calorie density (a high amount of calories for a small amount of volume)
- High in fat content
- High in sugar in liquid form

My suggestion is to choose fast-food options high in fiber (it exists!) that have a lower calorie density and a lower fat content and completely avoid sugar in liquid form when eating fast food. This means choosing fast food restaurants that have these types of offerings.

Do commercials for junk food make you eat more?

Let's start off by agreeing that the majority of food commercials targeting children are for junk foods—foods high in fat, sugar or salt and low in nutritional value. And if you've ever wondered if watching advertisements for assorted types of processed food products encourages children to eat more, some research suggests your suspicions are more than warranted.

Researchers from the University of Liverpool in the United Kingdom exposed 60 children, between the ages of 9 and 11, of varying weights, to both food advertisements and toy advertisements, followed by a cartoon and free food.

More food was eaten after the food advertisements than after the commercials for toys. Interestingly, the obese children increased their consumption of food the most (134 percent) compared to overweight children (101 percent) and normal weight children (84 percent).

I'm not surprised by these results. That is the whole point of food advertising, isn't it? To encourage consumption of the product? If it didn't work, why would food and beverage companies continue to spend millions on advertising? It does appear, though, that obese and overweight children are particularly vulnerable to this, and that in itself is alarming and worth noting to appropriate government agencies.

We can take junk food advertising out of our lives by limiting television viewing. Certain shows seem to attract more junk-food commercials more than others, so take note, parents, and discourage the viewing of these shows whenever possible. There are high-tech alternatives out there as well that help eliminate exposure to commercials, such as TIVO (which you can use to fast forward through commercials) or the use of show or movie DVDs.

Basically, to take the junk out of junk food, we need to choose foods and products with whole or real foods as often as possible and that contain less of certain ingredients such as sugar, high fructose corn syrup, milled grains, and partially hydrogenated oil.

Chapter 3

Everything You Ever Wanted to Ask Your Dietitian

Diet and type 2 diabetes

You've got questions about your diet and diabetes, and, hopefully, I've got answers for you. This chapter isn't meant to substitute for consulting with a dietitian or Certified Diabetes Educator (CDE) and working with them to fine tune your diet and lifestyle to normalize your blood sugars. It's designed to be a helpful compliment to working with them. If, after you read this chapter, you still have questions on food, diet, and diabetes, write them down as they pop into your mind and bring that list with you the next time you see your dietitian or CDE.

Q: Do you have a list of foods I cannot eat?

No—there isn't a list of foods you absolutely cannot eat. All foods, in smaller serving sizes, can be worked into a particular eating plan. If dietitians tell you that you can't have something anymore, it will only make you feel deprived and angry, and you will only want to have that food more. You ultimately decide what to eat. And it is you that will learn to associate certain foods, in certain amounts and in certain combinations, with higher blood sugars in your body.

Q: Are there any foods that might help someone with type 2 diabetes?

Studies support the importance of including whole grains, fruits, vegetables, and low-fat dairy in the diet of people with diabetes. An emphasis should be on balancing carbohydrates with monounsaturated fats and omega-3 fats when possible (these are what I like to call the "smart fats").

Here are some specific food suggestions that may help:

- **Fiber:** The chronic consumption of low amounts of fiber has been associated with an increased risk of type 2 diabetes as well as cancer, obesity, and heart disease.

- **Omega-3 fatty acids:** These may be especially helpful for people with type 2 diabetes who are at increased risk of heart disease.

- **Soy:** Soy may help people with diabetes control their blood sugar. Soy has been shown to make cells more responsive to insulin.

- **Buckwheat:** New research shows that extract of buckwheat lowered meal-related blood sugar levels by 12–19 percent when given to rats.

- **Moderate protein:** High protein intake causes the kidneys to work harder, which may damage kidney function over the long term, and people with diabetes are at increased risk of kidney disease.

- **Cinnamon:** The results of one study of 60 people suggests that less than half a teaspoon of ground cinnamon a day reduces blood sugar in people with type 2 diabetes. (*Diabetes Care* 26 [2003]: 3215–8)

- **Ground flaxseed:** There is some research suggesting there are health benefits for people with diabetes. (More on flaxseed in Chapter 4.)

- **A glass of wine:** With dinner, a glass may help lower fasting blood sugar in some people with diabetes, suggests a new Israeli study. The participants with the higher hemoglobin A1c levels saw the biggest reductions in fasting blood sugar. Along with potential health benefits, wine also brings 100 calories to the table, so you may need to trade these calories with another carbohydrate-rich food at dinner, because 100 calories are equal to about 25 grams of carbohydrate, higher doses of alcohol can be dangerous. Before starting any amount of alcohol consumption, you should talk with your doctor or dietitian. (Shai, I et al., "Glycemic Effects of Moderate Alcohol Intake Among Patients with Type 2 Diabetes." *Diabetes Care*, 30 [December 2007]: 3011–3016)

- **Nopal:** Also known as the prickly pear and a member of the cactus family, nopal may help lower blood glucose when it is cooked (not raw). Nopal may help decrease carbohydrate absorption, thanks to its high amount of fiber and pectin (soluble fiber). More research needs to be conducted, but the amount suggested as helpful when eaten with meals is at least 3.5 ounces of broiled nopal stems.

Q: I have a sweet tooth. Can I still eat some of my favorite desserts?

No one wants to be told they can't have something—especially sugar. It only makes you want it more. And there is no reason why people with diabetes can't have sugar, as long as they keep a few things in mind. Bread and several other starches actually have almost the same effect on blood sugar, in some people, as refined sugar does. But if the sugar-containing meal actually contains more carbohydrates than your meal plan suggests (worked out with your Certified Diabetes Educator), your blood sugar levels will likely go up.

With sugary foods, the rule is moderation, according to the American Diabetes Association. If you are managing your blood sugar well, then you may have some sugar, but you've got to play by a few rules:

- **Pay attention to portion sizes of sugary foods.** Keep servings moderate, such as a half cup of ice cream or three Oreo cookies.

- **Try to enjoy your dessert or high-sugar treat as part of a meal.** You will be less likely to overeat the treat if you have it with a meal, and the dessert will be less likely to send your blood sugar soaring if it's paired with other foods.

- **Substitute the sugar-containing food** for another carbohydrate-containing food in your personal diabetes meal plan. Otherwise you will not only increase the carbohydrates you're taking in, you'll also increase your calories.

- **Monitor your blood glucose routinely** so you'll be aware of any negative effects from the sugary food.

- **Taking a brisk walk** after the meal to burn some calories can also be helpful.

The lesson here: go ahead and eat cake, but make it a modest slice and have it with your meal. One last bit of advice: make sure these foods are truly satisfying, so you'll be happy with the moderate amounts.

Q: How can I do this without counting and measuring foods?

I don't like counting and measuring either. It automatically makes me feel "different" (and not in a good way) and, frankly, it can take the fun out of eating. I would strongly suggest doing some counting of carbohydrate, fat, and fiber grams every now and then, just to sort of "check in" with how you are eating. When you compare it to blood sugars, this can be a great tool for you and your dietitian or diabetes educator. But if you really can't bring yourself to do it, the only answer is to monitor, monitor, monitor (your blood sugar, that is). Monitor your blood sugar three to six times a day, study your normal diet and the resulting blood sugars, and soon you will know which foods or meals work best.

The foods that do cause high blood sugar may just need to be eaten in smaller amounts each time, combined with other foods, or coordinated with a change in medication or exercise just when that specific food/meal is eaten.

Q: Should I become vegetarian?

A total vegetarian diet can be high in carbohydrates, making normal blood sugars harder to achieve for some. If you choose to eat this way for other reasons, make sure you plan meals carefully to keep carbohydrates in check. You will need to depend heavily on plant foods that are higher in fat and protein, such as nuts, soybeans, and tofu, and plant foods rich in soluble fiber to help buffer the carbohydrate-induced rise in blood glucose. What might appeal more to most people is to eat not necessarily a "vegetarian diet," but to just plain eat more plant foods.

Q: I've heard there is a type of fiber that is good for people with type 2 diabetes. What is it?

Soluble fiber (fiber that is soluble, or dissolves, in water) seems to be a vital component of blood glucose control for many people. It is found in peas and beans, oats and oat bran, barley, and some fruits and other vegetables. Soluble fiber leaves the stomach slowly, so it makes you feel satisfied longer. I notice the feeling when I have beans with lunch, such as a bean burrito. (This is unusual because I am usually starving several hours after lunch.) Soluble fiber, which forms a gel within the intestinal tract, slows carbohydrate absorption and reduces the rise in blood glucose and insulin following the meal. Soluble fiber also has some disease-prevention benefits. Find out more about this in Chapter 4.

Q: Are the popular, very-high-protein, very-low-carbohydrate diets good for people with diabetes?

These diets aren't good for anyone, but they can be dangerous for people with type 2 diabetes. People with diabetes are already at high risk for kidney disease (diabetes increases the rate that the kidneys age) and excessive food protein and high blood pressure put even more stress on the kidneys. And people with diabetes do not have an increased need for protein than those without diabetes. Most high-protein diets are just fad diets in disguise—they aren't based on scientific and medical truths. Just think about it: Fruits, vegetables, and whole grains are some of the most nutritious foods on Earth, contributing vitamins, minerals, phytochemicals, and fiber. These foods are made up of mostly what? Carbohydrates. And while it is true that insulin is normally released into the blood stream when carbohydrates are eaten (in people without diabetes), the carbohydrates are stored as fat only if the amount of calories being eaten is greater than the amount needed by the body. So, carbohydrates don't automatically turn to fat unless you are eating too much.

Okay, so people say they have lost weight on these diets. The only thing that really counts is whether they were able to keep it off (and, in this respect, most people haven't been as lucky). People may lose weight on these diets not because they are low in carbohydrates, but because they tend to be low in calories. People do lose weight quickly, but it isn't fat they're losing right away; it's mostly body water. As you continue the diet, you will lose some fat pounds, but at the same time, you are losing muscle tissue.

When you eat too few carbohydrates, your body automatically starts to sacrifice its protein tissue (from major organs and muscles) for energy. And when you gain the weight back, it is likely as body fat, not muscle tissue. Over time, losing weight and gaining it back a few times causes you to get fatter and fatter and lose more and more muscle tissue. The liver and kidneys also have to work harder processing protein into energy than they would with carbohydrate.

Q: Are starchy foods, such as pasta, potatoes, and bread, fattening?

All of these foods are high in carbohydrate calories. Carbohydrates are only fattening when we eat more calories than our body needs. But this is also the case with foods high in protein and fat (*especially* fat). By including fruits and vegetables with these starches, we are more likely to keep our portions of these delicious starches reasonable. For example, when you fix pasta, add in some broccoli or carrots. When you make a sandwich with bread, have it with an apple, a wedge of melon, or a small bowl of fruit salad. With bread, you also have the opportunity to increase your daily fiber total by choosing bread that either contains whole grains or contains added soluble fiber.

Q: I'm confused. Is fat in food good or bad? I know it's bad for some diseases, but I also know it helps me control my blood sugars.

Over the past 15 years, needless to say, things have become much more complicated. Fat in food is feared; its mere presence has been known to inflict massive guilt on people. But the latest studies are showing us that some fats actually have a protective effect on our bodies in terms of heart disease and some cancers. They are also showing that there may not be one "right" amount of fat for all people; some people may fare better with more or less fat than others. Researchers are probably going to battle this out in the years to come, but, in the meantime, you're trying to get a better handle on your blood sugars, your weight, and your risk for heart disease.

I don't blame you for being confused. Most of us health professionals are trying to figure it all out too. Yes, having a moderate-fat diet (30 to 35 percent of calories from fat) seems to add up to better blood sugars for some people with type 2 diabetes, compared to a very low-fat diet (10 to 20 percent of calories from fat). The fat helps slow down digestion in general, and "paces" the introduction of glucose (from carbohydrates eaten) into the blood stream. For a variety of reasons, fat also helps some people feel more satisfied after a meal or snack.

The tricky part is knowing how much is enough for the diabetic benefits but not too much that it increases your risk for other chronic diseases and weight gain. I would try to stick around 30 to 35 percent calories from fat, and see what effect it has on your personal blood sugar, weight, and blood lipid levels. This way you could still have about 15 to 20 percent calories from protein, leaving around 45 to 55 percent calories from carbohydrate (hopefully mostly from whole grains, beans, fruits and vegetables).

As part of this moderate-fat eating plan you absolutely *must* turn to the more heart-protective fats—the omega-3 and omega-9 fatty acids and the monounsaturated fats—to make up most of the 35 percent. This means using canola oil and olive oil in cooking, choosing products that contain liquid canola oil or olive oil (non-hydrogenated), including flaxseed in your diet, enjoying a handful of nuts every now and then, and eating fish a couple times a week.

If you like eating out, these new rules could cramp your style. Most fast-food and regular restaurants do *not* use liquid canola and olive oil (except maybe an Italian or Mediterranean restaurant). You will learn more about eating out in Chapter 8.

Q: Do blood lipids tend to improve after people with type 2 diabetes switch to monounsaturated fats and omega-3 fatty acids?

Yes! Some people who achieve good blood sugar control on low fat/high carbohydrate diets unfortunately see their LDL ("bad") cholesterol and triglycerides increase. But after adding omega-3 fatty acids and monounsaturated fats to about 30 percent of calories from fat (or a little more), many people are able to improve their blood lipids without an increase in HgA1c (a blood test that, in essence, measures the 90-day average of blood sugars).

Q: The more I incorporate beans, which help my blood sugar, into my diet, the more gas I get. Is there anything I can do?

The fiber and some hard-to-digest complex carbohydrates in beans and legumes end up in the large intestine. The bacteria in the intestine then work on breaking down these substances, often giving off gas as a by-product, making you feel bloated. There are a few things you can do to minimize the gaseous effects of beans. Keep your serving of beans to about half a cup, to start with, and eat beans with a balanced meal (containing protein, fat, and carbohydrate). There are also a couple of over-the-counter products that claim to alleviate bean digestive distress, such as the products available at *www.beanogas.com* and *www.bean-zyme.com*.

Q: What are bad and good cholesterol?

A high level of LDL cholesterol in the blood increases the risk of fatty deposits forming in the arteries, increasing the risk of heart attack. That's how LDL has gotten its nickname as the "bad" cholesterol. Elevated levels of HDL cholesterol, on the other hand, seem to have a protective effect against heart disease, which is why it is fondly referred to as "good" cholesterol. One recent study revealed that even in the participants with optimal LDL cholesterol levels (below 70 mg/dL), those with the highest amount of HDL cholesterol levels were at less risk for major cardiovascular events compared to those with the lowest amount (*New England Journal of Medicine* Sept. 27, 2007).

What about total serum (blood) cholesterol levels? Many people think lowering *food* cholesterol is the most important step toward lowering *blood* cholesterol. Actually, eating less saturated fat has a stronger effect on lowering blood cholesterol levels. Some studies, though, have found that eating cholesterol increases the risk of heart disease, even if it doesn't increase blood cholesterol levels.

Q: Is there anything I can do to lower my blood lipid levels?

The complete answer to this question could fill an entire book or at least a chapter! But here's the short version.

Tips to lower high serum cholesterol

General suggestions include cutting back on fat (especially saturated fat and trans fats) and dietary cholesterol within reason, while eating more fruits, vegetables, and foods rich in soluble fiber (such as oats and beans). Here are some specific suggestions:

- Eating whole grains when possible and limiting simple sugars may be helpful.

- The Portfolio Plan, which includes soy protein, almonds, plant sterol-enriched margarines, and soluble fiber rich foods (oats, barley, psyllium, and vegetables such as okra and eggplant), has shown cholesterol-lowering benefits. The eating plan was developed by University of Toronto and research with the plan has tested the combination of four cholesterol-lowering foods. It can be found at *http://portfolioeatingplan.com*.

- Green tea's abundant antioxidants may also lower total cholesterol by increasing intestinal excretion of cholesterol and bile acids (through your stool).

Tips to lower LDL cholesterol

- According to the Portfolio Plan, reductions in bad cholesterol result from diets containing almonds and diets that are either low in saturated fat or high in viscous fibers (fiber that tends to be "sticky" in the intestinal tract), soy protein, or plant sterols.

- You can cut out a lot of saturated fat and trans fat from your diet by limiting full-fat dairy products, higher-fat meats, poultry skin, stick butter and margarine, commercially made cookies, crackers, and fast-food french fries.

- Eating a vegetarian diet that includes cholesterol-lowering foods (such as soy milk, soy burgers, oats, nuts, bean soup, and fruits and vegetables, which have all been individually found to lower cholesterol levels) may lower lipid levels as much as some medications (in one study, after one month, LDL levels fell by 29 percent, a drop similar to that seen with some statin drugs).

- Some studies have suggested that ground flaxseed, about four tablespoons a day, can lower LDL cholesterol from 9 to 18 percent and total blood cholesterol up to 9 percent. More clinical studies need to be done on ground flaxseed to confirm these positive effects, but there are so many other health benefits to a daily ground flaxseed regimen, that this seems to be the icing on the heart-healthy cake! For more tips, tricks, and recipes with ground flaxseed, check out my book, *The Flax Cookbook*.

Tips to lower triglycerides

- Limit saturated fat and trans fats and replace them with monounsaturated fats such as olive oil, canola oil, and most nuts.

- Cut back on refined carbohydrates such as sweets, soft drinks, and white bread.

- Limit alcoholic drinks to no more than one a day for women and two a day for men. People with diabetes should check with their doctor before consuming any amount of alcohol.

- Ground flaxseed may contribute to lowering triglyceride levels.

- Maintain a healthy weight and exercise regularly.

- People with diabetes who also have high triglycerides and high LDLs benefit from including more monounsaturated fats (olive oil, canola oil, and avocado) and slightly fewer carbohydrates.

- People with diabetes may benefit from eating fish twice a week. If you don't like fish, you might consider discussing fish oil capsules (one to three grams a day) with your doctor.

Tips to lower C-reactive protein

A high level of this protein can signal blood vessel inflammation and a greater likelihood of a rupture.

- Eat salmon, albacore tuna, sardines, walnuts, and ground flaxseed for omega-3 fatty acids.

- C-reactive protein was also lowered in two Portfolio studies in which people consistently consumed four key foods: soy protein, plant sterol-ester enriched margarine, almonds, and high soluble fiber foods.

- Maintain a healthy weight and exercise regularly.

Q: How and why do certain foods raise blood sugars more than others do? I find that pizza, for example, causes higher blood sugars than candy.

The foods we eat contain different amounts and combinations of carbohydrate, protein, and/or fat. Vegetable oils contain all fat and granulated sugar contains all carbohydrate. Other foods contain two or three of these. All of the grams of the digestible carbohydrates we eat convert to glucose, while about half of the protein and 10 percent of the fat grams we eat converts to glucose after digestion.

Carbohydrates, protein, and fat show their peak effect on blood glucose at different times after a meal, too:

- **Simple sugars:** Peak 15 to 30 minutes after the meal.
- **Complex carbohydrates:** Peak one to one and a half hours after the meal.
- **Protein:** Peaks three to four hours after the meal.
- **Fat:** Peaks three hours after the meal.

How a particular food affects your blood glucose has to do, in part, with the combination of carbohydrate, protein, and fat in the food and the portion size you eat. How quickly the food is absorbed (and how quickly it affects blood glucose levels) also depends on factors such as the physical form of the food, whether the food is cooked, and what blood glucose levels were before the meal. One trick all people with diabetes have up their sleeves is dietary fiber. Dietary fiber, which is not digested by the body, causes other carbohydrates in the meal to be digested and absorbed more slowly, encouraging lower blood sugars.

However, people respond differently to carbohydrates. The same meal eaten by different people might have varying effects on blood glucose levels. In some people, insulin becomes less effective after they eat high-animal-fat meals. This can also bring on high blood sugars. The only way to know for sure how your blood sugar responds to a particular meal is to test your blood sugar before and two hours after the meal.

Q: What are the meals and foods that encourage higher blood sugars, in some people, than would be normally expected?

Some health professionals call this "the pizza effect," so you can guess what is at the top of this list—pizza. Other foods that cause many people problems:

- Chinese food in general and chow mein in particular.
- Ramen noodles.
- Bagels eaten plain (even one bagel can cause a problem for some). Start with half a bagel and eat it with some peanut butter or light cream cheese.
- Fried foods, such as fried chicken and french fries.
- Granola cereal. Start with a quarter of a cup.
- Pasta. Try a 1-cup serving of cooked 100-percent durum wheat semolina pasta, and start the meal with a soup or salad.
- High animal protein/fat meals, including those with lots of cheese, such as a big cheese omelet served with sausage or bacon, or a big steak dinner served with french fries.
- Cold breakfast cereals.
- Baked potatoes.
- Watermelon and other melons.

Q: Are there any foods that can help prevent high blood sugar, when they are paired with foods that usually cause high blood sugar?

Adding plant foods that contribute some fat and/or protein to the meal (nuts, soy foods, olive and canola oil, flaxseed, avocado) seems to help minimize high blood sugars from notorious high carbohydrate meals. But if you have a meal high in animal fat that usually brings on high blood sugars (pizza, high-fat breakfasts, etc.), loading up on fiber (soluble fiber in particular) about 10 minutes before you start the meal may help. Higher soluble fiber plant foods will also help minimize high blood sugars from high carbohydrate meals. As an appetizer, before you eat the entrée, try:

- A green salad with kidney beans and raw vegetables.
- A cup of vegetable or bean soup.
- A small serving of oat bran or oatmeal (before a problematic breakfast).
- Other high soluble fiber vegetables (see Chapter 4).
- Other high soluble fiber grain foods (see Chapter 4).
- Psyllium seed foods and supplements. (Powders without intestinal stimulants are available. Pysllium is also added to a couple of breakfast cereals.)

Q: Why do I seem to have higher blood sugars after high-fat meals instead of high-carbohydrate meals?

Some people seem to have high blood sugars after meals particularly high in animal fats, such as bacon and eggs, or pizza topped with sausage and pepperoni. Some researchers think that in some people (particularly certain ethnicities such as Asians,

Pacific Islanders, and African Americans) insulin becomes less effective after meals laden in animal fat. If you notice this happens with you, try having smaller portions of the fatty foods and add in some plant foods (fruits, vegetables, and grains, especially those rich in soluble fiber) and see if it makes a difference. Instead of bacon, eggs, and hash browns, try one sausage link, one egg, and pancakes or a bowl of oatmeal. Trade in your four slices of "meat lover's" pizza for a couple slices of "vegetable lover's" pizza plus a green salad with kidney beans and an olive oil vinaigrette, or a nice cup of vegetable or bean soup.

Q: What is the percentage of carbohydrates, fat, and protein that seems to help most people with type 2 diabetes control blood sugars?

According to Certified Diabetes Educators who I spoke with, about one-third of the people with type 2 diabetes tend to do better with an eating plan with 35 to 40 percent calories from fat (using mostly monounsaturated fats), while two-thirds tend to fair best with a 25 to 30 percent calories from fat. But there are many other food factors, other than the percent of fat or carbohydrates, that can influence blood sugar control, such as total fiber/soluble fiber and whether proteins and fats come mostly from vegetable sources.

Q: What is a good breakfast if your blood sugars tend to be high in the morning?

Many people with type 2 diabetes have trouble with morning blood sugars, not necessarily because of what they ate for breakfast, but because their "wake-up" blood sugars started high. Many people tend to be more resistant to insulin in the morning and carbohydrates are generally less tolerated at breakfasts than at other meals during the day. Start by fixing yourself a nice balanced breakfast, with carbohydrate, protein, and fat. You can do this by adding nuts to cereal and muffins. Some people don't mind adding plain soy milk or almond milk to their cereals in the morning. If you are having pancakes, serve up a couple slices of turkey bacon or Canadian bacon. If you are having a bagel, add a slice of cheese, a tablespoon or two of peanut butter, or two tablespoons of light cream cheese. Enjoy an egg-substitute omelet filled with vegetables!

Q: What about wine? Does one glass at dinner help lower blood sugars?

A glass of red wine with dinner does seem to encourage lower blood sugars for some people, but it is very individual. For others, the opposite can happen—blood sugars seem to rise later that night. Sweeter wines tend to bring on higher blood sugars, so people tend to do better with red wines and drier wines. If you do have a glass of wine with dinner, check your blood sugar before bed, and, if you can, try testing your blood sugar at 2 or 3 a.m. every now and then. Let your Certified Diabetes Educator know if it seems to help normalize your blood sugar or elevate it.

Q: What artificial or alternative sweeteners should I buy in products or add to food if I want some sweeteners without adding carbohydrates?

Artificial sweeteners come in handy if you are trying to reduce your calories from sugar, if you have diabetes and are trying to maintain normal blood sugar, and if you happen to like the taste of diet soda because regular soda is too darn sweet.

Can they really help with weight loss? According to a study by Dutch researchers, artificial sweeteners may have a pivotal role in our weight-loss and weight-maintenance plans. After reviewing many recent studies, they noted that the use of aspartame was associated with improved weight maintenance after a year. When artificially sweetened beverages were substituted for regular, sweetened beverages (and calories were not restricted), people ended up eating fewer calories and weighing less, according to the results of two short-term studies (*American Journal of Clinical Nutrition,* February 1997).

Another Harvard Medical School study reported similar results in 1997. They assigned obese women to either consume or eliminate aspartame-sweetened foods for 16 weeks of a weight-reduction program. What happened? The women who were consuming the artificial sweetener lost significantly more weight overall and regained significantly less weight during the maintenance and follow-up phase (*American Journal of Clinical Nutrition,* February 1997).

I still wouldn't go crazy for alternative sweeteners, though, and consume unlimited amounts. I think moderation might be in order here, too. Although not scientifically proven yet, some experts suspect, and I agree, that artificially sweetened food and drink may psych out our bodies, so to speak, by telling our brains that something sweet is coming (as our taste buds sense the sweetness as we chew and swallow) and yet the body isn't getting the sugar calories it's expecting. This might, in some people, make them crave some real carbohydrate as a response to the unrequited consumption of simple carbohydrate.

Q: Which artificial sweetener is right for me?

With so many artificial sweeteners out there these days, how do you know which one to buy? Here's how they differ, and the pros and cons of each type.

Sucralose (Splenda)

Splenda contains the artificial sweetener sucralose, along with maltodextrin, which adds bulk so Splenda can be substituted cup-for-cup for sugar in recipes. Sucralose is 600 times sweeter than sugar. To make sucralose, they take a cane sugar molecule and substitute three hydrogen-oxygen groups with three chlorine atoms. After experimenting with Splenda in baking recipes, I have found the results are usually successful when I use half sugar and half Splenda.

Pros:

- Sucralose has no calories, is not considered a carbohydrate by the body, and has no effect on blood sugar levels.

- You can bake with Splenda. Heat doesn't lessen the sweet taste.

- When it comes to baking and cooking, Splenda appears to be the best sweetener for the job.

- Of all the artificial sweeteners, Splenda has caused the least controversy from watchdog or consumer groups.

- After more than 110 studies (including animal and human studies), the FDA concluded that sucralose was shown to have no toxic or carcinogenic effects, no DNA altering, and it does not pose reproductive or neurological risks to humans.

Cons:

- The bulking agents used in Splenda can add around 12 calories per tablespoon of the mixture (although the package does not list these calories).

- Splenda can change the texture in baking recipes and can add an "artificial" taste when used as the only sweetener in the recipe.

- Some critics claim that preliminary animal research has linked Splenda to organ damage.

Saccharin (Sweet'N Low)

Saccharin, which is 300 times sweeter than sugar, is an organic molecule made from petroleum. After bladder cancer was found in male lab rats that were fed huge amounts of saccharin, the FDA proposed a ban on saccharin in 1977. But no ban was enacted, and the warning label on saccharin was dropped in 2000.

Pros:

- Heat doesn't affect its sweetness.

Cons:

- Since 1981, government reports have listed saccharin as an "anticipated human carcinogen." Although studies of heavy saccharin users don't support any link with cancer, certain subgroups, such as male heavy smokers, may be at increased risk.
- The American Medical Association's Council on Scientific Affairs suggests that parents and caregivers limit young children's intake of saccharin, because little information is available on how it might affect them.
- Because saccharin can cross the placenta, the Council on Scientific Affairs suggests that women use saccharin carefully during pregnancy.

Aspartame (NutraSweet and Equal)

You would never guess that one of the most popular artificial sweeteners is actually a combination of two amino acids, phenylalanine and aspartic acid, which are then combined with methanol. It is 180–200 times sweeter than sugar.

Some 70 percent of our aspartame intake is from soft drinks. The FDA has set the acceptable daily intake (ADI, the estimated amount a person can safely consume every day over a lifetime) at 50 mg per kilogram of body weight. For most of us, this probably translates to about four 12-ounce cans of diet soda or nine 8-ounce glasses of fruit drink made from powder.

Pros:

- Each gram of aspartame has four calories, but it adds almost no calories to foods or drinks because we need only a tiny amount of aspartame to mimic the sweetness of sugar.

- The FDA has evaluated aspartame use in food and beverages 26 times since the sweetener was first approved in 1981. In 1996, the FDA approved its use as a general-purpose sweetener in foods and beverages.

- In 1985, the AMA's Council on Scientific Affairs concluded that "available evidence suggests that consumption of aspartame by normal humans is safe and is not associated with serious adverse health effects."

- Use of aspartame within the FDA guidelines appears safe for pregnant women.

Cons:

- People born with a condition called phenylketonuria cannot metabolize the amino acid phenylalanine.

- Aspartame breaks down in liquids that are exposed to heat, so we can't bake or cook with it.

- Some people claim they have had allergic reactions to aspartame, ranging from skin reactions to respiratory problems, but this has been difficult to confirm in studies.

- Some people have reported central nervous system side effects, such as headaches, dizziness, and mood changes, after consuming aspartame. But after reviewing 600 of these complaints, the Center for Disease Control concluded there was no association. (The Environmental Nutrition newsletter later reported that the CDC was leaving open the possibility that a small group of people is very sensitive to aspartame.)

Acesulfame-K (Sunette or Sweet One)

Acesulfame-K (the "K" refers to mineral potassium) is 200 times sweeter than sugar. It is approved by the FDA as a tabletop sweetener and an additive to desserts, confections, and alcoholic beverages.

Pros:

- It doesn't increase the risk of cancer, according to government agencies.
- It doesn't affect blood-sugar levels.
- It can be used in cooking and baking.
- It isn't broken down by the body during digestion and is excreted from the body unchanged.
- Combining it with other artificial sweeteners can increase the overall sweetness and decrease the bitter taste.
- The use of acesulfame-K within FDA guidelines appears safe for pregnant women.

Cons:

- When used on its own, this sweetener can have a bitter taste.
- The Washington-based consumer group Center for Science in the Public Interest believes the safety tests on

acesulfame-K were poorly conducted and did not properly assess the sweetener's cancer-causing potential.

Sugar Alcohols (sorbitol, mannitol, maltitol, and xylitol)

These sugar alcohols are found in nature (in plant foods such as fruits and berries) and are also commercially made for use as sweeteners. They are absorbed slowly, and part of them isn't absorbed at all, which is why consuming larger amounts can lead to diarrhea, gas, and bloating. About 50 percent of the sugar alcohols convert to glucose, so keep in mind that they still have an effect on blood sugar, but to a lesser degree than sugar.

Pros:
- Sorbitol has received the "Generally Recognized as Safe" designation from the FDA.

Cons:
- Some people experience a laxative effect if they consume more than 49 grams of sorbitol or more than 19 grams of mannitol.

The bottom line on artificial sweeteners

So which one do you choose when you want to add alternative sweetener to a food or beverage? That's really up to you as you weigh the pros and cons of each, but it seems many of the Certified Diabetes Educators I spoke with suggest Splenda to their patients as the alternative sweetener of choice.

But everything in moderation. We can't just put all our weight-loss eggs in the artificial-sweetener basket. In other words, don't expect that simply switching to sugar-free products will help you lose weight and keep it off. This should be just one piece of your plan to start living healthy by eating right, avoiding overeating, and exercising as much as possible.

Chapter 4

The 10 Food Steps to Freedom

True, you need to work out an individualized eating plan with your dietitian or Certified Diabetes Educator, because what works best to normalize your blood sugars may be different for someone else. But there are 10 things all people with type 2 diabetes can do to improve their health, reduce their risk of heart disease and other health risks, and to make normal blood sugars more likely. Following these 10 steps will bring you one giant step closer to feeling better, having normal blood sugars, and living a longer, healthier life.

Food Step

Step #1: Make fiber a part of almost every meal.

Fiber is the part in plant foods that humans can't digest. Because we can't digest it, it makes it all the way through the mouth to the stomach, then through the small and large intestines without being absorbed, and out the other end. But even though it isn't absorbed, it does all sorts of great stuff for our bodies.

The most important thing about fiber

Research shows that fiber helps reduce the rapid rise in blood sugar that tends to take place after eating foods containing carbohydrates. It does this by slowing down their digestion. This could help blunt the impact of eating carbohydrates on people at risk for diabetes!

There are two types of fiber. There is insoluble fiber, which doesn't dissolve in water and contributes "roughage" or "bulk" to our intestinal tract. It acts like scrubbers, pushing food along and helping to clean the intestinal wall as it passes through. This is the type of fiber that is thought to help treat and prevent diverticulosis (a condition in which small pouches form in the colon wall and can become infected) and is linked to reducing the risk of constipation and colon cancer. It is possible that the fiber latches onto potential carcinogens within the intestines and carries them out of the body.

The second type of fiber is particularly important if you have type 2 diabetes: soluble fiber. Soluble fiber is different from the other type of fiber because it dissolves in water and becomes almost gel-like. Soluble fiber does appear to lower total serum cholesterol and LDL cholesterol levels (the higher your cholesterol levels, the more it will help lower it). It also helps regulate blood sugars. Because soluble fiber helps regulate blood sugars, high-fiber diets have been reported to:

- Lower postprandial blood sugar. (It may even improve glucose control in the meals immediately following.)
- Decrease glucose in the urine.
- Decrease insulin needs and increase tissue sensitivity to insulin.
- Reduce levels of atherosclerosis-promoting blood lipids.

It's soluble fiber, in particular, that may help lessen the potential increase in blood triglycerides and other blood fats seen in some diabetics on a high-carbohydrate diet.

One study showed that a high-fiber eating plan reduced insulin requirements by 75 percent in people with type 2 diabetes. Some people were able to get off insulin completely. There is one catch: soluble fiber helps lower your glucose level *after* meals, and, to a lesser extent, your wake-up glucose reading. But this is still super-helpful because we spend most of our 24-hour day in a post-meal state, right? How much total fiber are we talking about? A stiff daily dose of about 30 grams of fiber.

In another study on men with diabetes, this one from UCLA, a combination of a higher-fiber, low-fat diet resulted in significant reductions in fasting glucose and insulin levels as well as in body mass index and all serum lipids (*Diabetes Research Clinical Practice* Sept. 2006 73[3]: 249–59).

How much fiber do we need to get our heart disease prevention benefits? In one study, men who ate more than 25 grams of fiber per day (soluble and insoluble), reduced their risk of heart disease by 36 percent, compared to men who ate less than 15 grams of fiber daily. Does this sound impossible? With the right tips and recipes, and maybe a small hill of beans, some of us can hit this mark on most days.

How does soluble fiber work its magic?

Fiber slows down the absorption of other nutrients eaten at the same meal, including carbohydrates. This slowing down may help prevent peaks and valleys in your blood sugars. It has also been suggested that higher-fiber meals improve your body sensitivity to insulin, so it may reduce the insulin requirements in insulin-treated type 2 diabetics.

As it passes through the intestines, soluble fiber holds onto anything it can and carries it out of the body. One of the things we know it holds onto is bile (digestive juices that the body produces using cholesterol from the body), so our body has to keep making more bile, using more cholesterol. This reduces blood cholesterol levels. Everybody responds differently, but, for some people, combining soluble fiber with a low-fat eating plan can mean serum cholesterol reductions of 50 points or more.

Getting fiber at almost every meal

The problem is that the typical American diet is anything but high in fiber. "White" grain is the American mode of operation; we eat a muffin or bagel made with white flour in the morning, have our hamburger on a white bun, then have white rice with our dinner. The more refined, or "whiter," the grain-based food, the lower the fiber.

To get some fiber into almost every meal takes effort. Start by:

• Eating plenty of fruits and vegetables. Just eating five servings a day of fruits and vegetables (something we should do anyway) will get you to about five grams of soluble fiber. See Step #6 for more on fruits and vegetables.

• Including some beans and bean products in your diet. A half cup of cooked beans will add about two grams of soluble fiber to your day.

• Switching to whole grains whenever possible.

Thanks to all the wonderful whole-grain blend pastas now on the market, higher-fiber pasta is now a way of life in the Magee house. Just switch where you can but know that the more you switch from refined-grain products to the higher-fiber whole-grain foods, the better off you will be with your health in general and, most likely, with your diabetes.

Q: Where can you find soluble fiber?

Most plant foods contain some insoluble fiber and some soluble fiber. About one-quarter to one-third of the total amount of fiber in plants is the soluble type, but some plant foods have more than others. The following foods are some of the richest sources of soluble fiber.

- **Beans:** One half-cup cooked kidney beans, butterbeans, canned baked beans, blackbeans, navy beans, lentils, pinto beans, great northern beans, chick peas or garbanzo, split peas, and lima beans. Some of the soluble fiber dissolves in the liquid of canned beans, so if you are making a soup or stew, just stir the liquid in.

- **Oats and oat bran:** One-half cup dry oat bran contributes three grams of soluble fiber, and 1 cup of cooked oatmeal contains about 2 grams of soluble fiber. One packet of instant oatmeal contributes 1 gram of soluble fiber.

- **Barley:** This grain has been enjoyed in other parts of the world for hundreds of years. In America, you sometimes find it in soups. Even pearl barley, which has been milled, still contributes 1.8 grams of soluble fiber per three-quarter-cup cooked serving.

- **Some fruits:** Apples; mango; plums; kiwi; pears; blackberries; strawberries; raspberries; peaches; citrus fruits, including oranges and grapefruits (you'll get the most soluble fiber if you include the "pulp" and membranes dividing the fruit into sections); dried fruits, including dried apricots, prunes, and figs.

- **Some vegetables:** Artichoke, celery root, sweet potato, parsnip, turnip, acorn squash, potato with skin, brussel sprouts, cabbage, green peas, broccoli, carrots, french-style green beans, cauliflower, asparagus, and beets.

• **Psyllium seed products:** One rounded kitchen teaspoon of most psyllium products will give you about 3 grams of soluble fiber.

Give it time and lots of water

Most people's bodies seem to adjust to more fiber in their diet within about six weeks. While your body is "adjusting," you may notice a little uninvited gas. To minimize the side effects (diarrhea, abdominal pain, and flatulence) increase your fiber *slowly* and drink plenty of water (which you should be doing anyway). Soluble fiber, especially, absorbs water like a sponge, so drink up!

You can also try Beano or Beanzyme pills, which are found in your local drugstore or on the Internet. They contain an enzyme that, when taken along with beans, cabbage, broccoli, and other vegetables, helps reduce the side effects. For a handful of great bean recipes, see Chapter 6. For lists of higher-fiber cereals, see Chapter 7.

The high-fiber bonus for calorie watchers

Both fiber types help us feel fuller faster when they are part of the meal, discouraging overeating. When people eat meals higher in fiber, they tend to eat less. One study found that people ate smaller lunches after eating high-fiber breakfasts. Why? Fiber lowers insulin, and insulin helps stimulate your appetite. And fiber seems to help make you feel full.

There is also some evidence that fiber can help cut calories by blocking the digestion of some of the fat, protein, or carbohydrates eaten at the same time. Either way, eating fiber is a good thing if you are overweight.

Food Step

Step #2: Count carbohydrates and know your ideal carbohydrate budget per meal.

Every Certified Diabetes Educator I spoke with agreed that it is essential to determine your carbohydrate budget per meal to ensure you are hitting your carbohydrate budget. You can compare your carbohydrate intake at a meal to your blood sugar levels one-and-a-half to two hours after the meal, to get a better idea of how to adjust your carbohydrate budget for that particular meal to gain normal blood sugars.

It isn't that carbohydrates are bad. It's just that you need to know what amount of carbohydrates your body can tolerate (at different times of the day) given your body, medication, and exercise schedule. Also, keep in mind, many Certified Diabetes Educators believe it is actually more important to know your carbohydrate budget per meal or snack than it is to know what it is per day.

Your individualized carbohydrate budget

If you are not on insulin, try focusing on keeping the amount of carbohydrate consistent throughout the day. If you are on insulin, decide with your Certified Diabetes Educator how much carbohydrate to aim for at meals. Create a carbohydrate budget, a certain daily and meal total of grams of carbohydrate. If you go over or under these amounts, you may need to adjust your insulin according to your Certified Diabetes Educator's instructions.

Figuring out your carbohydrate budget

No food is off limits! It's more about learning to spend your carbohydrate budget wisely throughout the day. One of the reasons to focus on counting grams of carbohydrate is because they have the fastest effect on increasing your blood sugar levels. Your Certified Diabetes Educator or dietitian will consider the following factors when calculating your suggested carbohydrate budget:

- Your weight and height.
- Whether or not weight loss is recommended by your health team.
- When and how much exercise you tend to get. (Physical activity acts a bit like insulin in your body and will help lower your blood sugar.)
- Your diabetes medication or insulin and when you take it.
- Other medical issues, such as elevated blood lipids.

Q: How low can you go with carbohydrates?

The key for many people with type 2 diabetes, in terms of avoiding high blood sugars with diet, is avoiding those common high-carbohydrate, low-fiber meals. Put another way, this means eating meals with a more moderate amount of carbohydrate. This can help some people lose weight and gain better blood sugars. However, it doesn't need to be as low in carbohydrates as the Atkins diet, according to Rosemary Yurczyk and other dietitians I spoke with, who work day-to-day helping people with type 2 diabetes. People tend to want to view things as black or white, good or bad; and when the true answer lies in practicing moderation, then that becomes the tricky part for many people.

Here are answers to some questions I posed to Certified Diabetes Educator extrodinaire, Rosemary Yurczyk, MS, RD, CDE, in March 2008.

Q: What are the guidelines used as a carbohydrate budget starting point for people with type 2 diabetes to work from?

Rosemary likes to recommend about 30–60 grams per meal for women and about 60–90 grams per meal for men. This seems like a big range but the amount that often ends up working for her clients depends on their weight, blood sugar goals, exercise, type of medicine, current eating habits, etc. This is why working closely with a Certified Diabetes Educator to find your personalized carbohydrate budget is a great idea.

A starting point for women

"If you figure that many women trying to lose weight may need to consume about 1,500 calories per day, and 50 percent of their calories come from carbohydrate, that is about 187 grams of carbohydrate per day or about 60 grams per meal," explains Yurczyk. That's for three meals a day, and, if you are using a four-meal-a-day schedule, it works out to around 47 grams of carbohydrate per meal or snack.

For her patients that want to be on less medication and/or who have severe insulin resistance, Rosemary Yurczyk recommends trying a little less carbohydrate: 40 percent calories from carbohydrate. Given this guideline, our calculations for a 1,500 calories per day benchmark, work out to 150 grams of carbohydrate per day or about 50 grams per meal with three meals a day, or 38 grams of carbohydrate per meal with four meals or snacks a day.

A starting point for men

For a man trying to lose weight, the goal is closer to the 2,000 calorie a day benchmark; 50 percent calories from carbohydrate would translate to about 250 grams of carbohydrate per day, or about 80 grams of carbohydrate per meal for three meals a day. If you are using the four-meal-a-day schedule, it works out to around 60 grams of carbohydrate per meal or snack.

For her male patients that want to be on less medication and/ or who have severe insulin resistance, Rosemary Yurczyk recommends trying a little less carbohydrate: 40 percent calories from carbohydrate. Given this guideline, our calculations for a 2,000 calories per day benchmark work out to 200 grams of carbohydrate per day, or about 66 grams per meal with three meals a day, or 50 grams of carbohydrate per meal with four meals or snacks a day.

A piece of cake or a cup of rice

For the most part, if the amount of carbohydrate is the same, a serving of cake is a lot like a serving of rice, pasta, or bread. The effect on your blood sugars will be similar, particularly if it is eaten as part of a meal instead of by itself.

Here are some examples of what foods (and how much) add up to 25–30 grams of carbohydrate:

Food and serving size	Carb. (grams)	Fat (grams)	Fiber (grams)
applesauce, unsweetened	28	0.1	3
broccoli, cooked, 3 cups	25	1.6	14
brown rice, cooked, 2/3 cup	30	1.2	2.4
yellow cake, 1/15th of prepared cake from mix	29	9.6	0
chocolate cake with icing	28	8.5	1.5

Food and serving size	Carb.	Fat	Fiber
cookies, sandwich type, 4	28	8.2	1.2
ice cream, light, 2/3 cup	25	5	0
kidney beans, canned, 3/4 cup	31	1.8	9
oatmeal, homemade, 1 cup	25	2.3	4
orange juice, fresh, 8 oz	25	0	0
Raisin Bran cereal, 2/3 cup	30	1	4.7
Rice Krispies cereal, 1 1/4 cup	29	0	0
Snickers Bar, 1 1/2 ounces	26	9.5	1.3
strawberries, 2 1/2 cup sliced	29	1.5	6.4
watermelon, cubes, 2 1/2 cups	29	1.7	1
whole-wheat bagel, 1 (55 g)	31	0.8	5
whole-wheat bread, 2 slices	32	2.9	4.3
whole-wheat pasta, cooked	28	0.6	4
whole-wheat pita, 1	25	1.2	3.2
yogurt, low-fat fruit, 6 oz	32.5	2	0.2

Q: Is there a certain amount of moderate-sized meals per day that seems to work best for most type 2 diabetic patients?

Most of Rosemary's patients still eat three meals a day, plus a snack if needed in the afternoon. The most important thing to

Rosemary is that their food is distributed throughout the day and that they are eating about every four hours.

This might look like:

- Breakfast around 7 or 8 a.m.
- Lunch sometime around noon
- A small afternoon snack between 3 and 4 p.m.
- A light dinner around 6 or 7 p.m.
- Some wonderfully flavored decaf green tea (or other non-calorie or low-cal beverage that you enjoy) around 9 p.m.

Q: Is morning a particularly problematic time due to higher insulin resistance in the morning? What seems to work best at this time of day?

Increased hormones in the morning seem to increase insulin resistance for people with type 2 diabetes, according to Rosemary. Being vigilant about keeping track of the carbohydrate grams and fiber grams eaten at breakfast and the resultant blood sugars (in a journal) will help people understand what is the ideal number of carbohydrate and fiber grams for them first thing in the morning. This might be a time of day when you need to shoot for the lower amount of carbohydrates per meal (50 grams for women and 66 grams for men) and when you really want to reach that per meal fiber goal of seven to eight grams.

Q: How does fiber fit into your carbohydrate budget?

You can't talk about carbohydrates and type 2 diabetes, or carbohydrates and good health in general, without talking about fiber. Remember how having a good amount of fiber grams in your meals helps the body better manage the carbohydrate grams you are eating? Well, your carbohydrate budget will also have a fiber budget. Whereas the carbohydrate budget is there to make sure you aren't going over it, the fiber budget is there to make sure you aren't going below it. "I think people are way too low in their fiber intake," notes Rosemary.

Eating about 25 to 30 grams of fiber a day is a challenging but powerful goal, and this amount of fiber will benefit your body more ways than I can count, starting with better blood sugar levels and a happier colon. If you are eating four moderately sized meals a day, the desirable fiber amount per meal is in the ballpark of around seven grams. Now, that's not too scary, is it?

Don't forget to do the math

Because eating more fiber helps the body manage the carbohydrates in the meal better, many dietitians suggest their patients subtract the grams of fiber in the meal from the carbohydrate grams being eaten to give the "net" amount of carbohydrate grams.

In other words, if you ate 50 grams of carbohydrate in your meal and the meal also contains seven grams of fiber, your true or net amount of carbohydrates to subtract from your daily carbohydrate budget would be 43. Make sense?

There's weight-loss magic in the food diary

There's some magic in keeping a food diary; one recent study found it can double a person's weight loss! The researchers discovered that the more food records people kept, the more weight they lost. Published in the August 2008 issue of *American Journal of Preventive Medicine*, the study adds more evidence to the notion that the simple act of writing down what you eat encourages people to consume fewer calories. This is an added bonus for people with diabetes who are also trying to trim off a few extra pounds. (Hollis, J. F. et al. "Weight Loss During the Intensive Intervention Phase of the Weight-Loss Maintenance Trial." *American Journal of Preventative Medicine* 35, no. 2: 118–126)

Most of the commercial food diaries available leave a space only to tabulate grams of carbohydrate. I designed the following A Day at a Glance chart to help you tabulate grams of carbohydrate, plus grams of fat and fiber if desired. Knowing the grams of fat and fiber helps complete the picture for many people with diabetes. You might find that it's the really high-fat meals that cause you trouble, or you might find that a certain amount of fat grams seems to help normalize your blood sugars. You might discover that your blood sugars are better when your meal/snack contains a high-fiber food.

The A Day at a Glance chart includes a space to record how hungry you were when you ate. There is a space to record your blood sugar, your medication, the minutes and when you exercised. All this information will help you and your dietitian or diabetes educator fine-tune your eating plan.

A Day at a Glance

Blood Sugar Measurements

6 a.m. _____

8 a.m. _____

10 a.m. _____

12 p.m. _____

2 p.m. _____

4 p.m. _____

6 p.m. _____

8 p.m. _____

10 p.m. _____

12 a.m. _____

2 a.m. _____

Insulin or Oral Measurements (record units or number of tablets taken at what times)

6 a.m. _____

8 a.m. _____

10 a.m. _____

12 p.m. _____

2 p.m. _____

4 p.m. _____

6 p.m. _____

8 p.m. _____

10 p.m. _____

12 a.m. _____

2 a.m. _____

Activity (minutes)

6 a.m. _____

8 a.m. _____

10 a.m. _____

12 p.m. _____

2 p.m. _____

4 p.m. _____

6 p.m. _____

8 p.m. _____

10 p.m. _____

12 a.m. _____

2 a.m. _____

Meals/Snacks   Day:_____   Date: ___/___/___

meal/snack   carbs   fat   fiber   hunger level

_____

meal/snack   carbs   fat   fiber   hunger level

_____

meal/snack	carbs	fat	fiber	hunger level
meal/snack	carbs	fat	fiber	hunger level

(*Hunger level: 4 = very hungry, 3 = moderately hungry, 2 = somewhat hungry, 1 = not really hungry)

Step #3: Switch to smart carbohydrates and emphasize low-glycemic-load foods.

Food Step

Is the glycemic index, or GI, essentially, a number that says how much your blood sugar rises after you eat a particular food that contains carbohydrates, really the be-all, end-all to nutrition and health?

Well, not exactly.

High-GI foods, such as white bread and white rice, give you a quick blood-sugar boost that also fades quickly, leaving you hungry again. Lower-GI foods, such as whole grains, produce, and beans, keep you feeling full longer, because they cause your blood-sugar levels to rise more slowly.

I call the glycemic index a work in progress, because, while it is certainly one tool that can be considered when making food choices, it's not the only means to measure what you eat. That's because it's based on how blood sugar rises in response to one particular food, such as carrots or rice. But we don't sit down to just a bowl of carrots or a plate of rice, do we? We eat foods together, as dishes and meals. The presence of fat or fiber in a meal also influences how quickly our bodies metabolize the carbohydrates. So do some other factors, such as how long noodles are cooked, or how finely grain is ground. For example, slightly undercooked noodles are absorbed more slowly and have a lower GI, and the more finely a grain is ground, the more quickly its carbohydrates are absorbed.

Here's where the controversy kicks in. Researchers and experts continue to disagree on whether low-GI foods lead to weight loss, lower blood sugar levels, and/or a reduced risk of heart disease and cancer compared with high-GI foods.

After reviewing the existing research, the American Institute for Cancer Research (AICR) concluded: "Due to insufficient evidence of clinical efficiency and persistent methodological concerns regarding how glycemic index values are determined, AICR cautions the public not to make dietary changes based solely on this interesting but still unproven concept." Enter a potentially more useful tool: the glycemic load.

The better way to measure

The glycemic load (GL) is like the glycemic index, in that the lower the number, the better the blood glucose response is predicted to be. But GL values allow comparisons of the likely glycemic effect of realistic serving sizes of the foods. So while carrots tend to have a somewhat high glycemic index, the glycemic load is actually low because it factors in the grams of carbohydrates for a realistic serving size.

What this means is that the glycemic index tells you how quickly a particular carbohydrate in food makes your blood sugar rise, but it doesn't take into account how many carbohydrates are found in a serving. That means that some healthy, but relatively lower-carbohydrate, foods—such as carrots—end up with a high GI number.

The glycemic load, meanwhile, takes the number of carbohydrates per serving into consideration along with the food's glycemic index. To find a food's glycemic load, you multiply its GI value by number of carbohydrates per serving.

Q: What influences the glycemic load and glycemic index?

Many factors help determine your body's glycemic response to a particular food, including:

- **Physical form, such as a whole apple vs. applesauce:** Mashing foods tends to give them a higher glycemic index/load.

- **Ripeness:** The riper the fruit, the higher its glycemic index.

- **Fiber:** Particularly viscous fiber, a type of soluble fiber found in oats, barley, and other foods. Generally, the higher the fiber, the lower the glycemic index/load.

- **Acidity:** The higher a food's acidity, the lower its glycemic index/load.

- **Processing:** The more processed or refined a food, generally, the higher its glycemic index/load will be. When a grain is in a more "whole" form, your body's digestive enzymes have a tougher time breaking it down, which lowers the glycemic response to it. There are some notable exceptions: pasta, and parboiled and basmati rice tend to have lower glycemic indexes, especially if they're not overcooked.

- **Whether protein and fat were eaten with the food:** The presence of high amounts of protein and fat will decrease the glycemic index/load.

The following foods, when eaten alone, even in large amounts, are not likely to cause a significant rise in blood sugar, because they contain little carbohydrate: meat, poultry, fish, avocados, salad vegetables, eggs, fish, and cheese.

The bottom line on glycemic load and glycemic index

I always look for the bottom line, and in the case of glycemic load, it tends to lead you to less-processed types of carbohydrate-rich foods, such as vegetables, fruits, whole grains, beans, and legumes. The truth is that there is plenty of evidence that a mostly plant-based diet can reduce your risk of diseases such as cancer, heart disease, and diabetes. And these foods tend to have lower glycemic index numbers. But we have yet to determine whether a low glycemic index diet is really what helps prevent disease, or whether this effect comes mostly from eating a healthful variety of foods.

Glycemic load and index values for common foods

Here are glycemic index (GI) and glycemic load (GL) values for some common foods. I have included their fiber content as well. Keep in mind that GI/GL is just one tool. Other aspects of food (such as its vitamin, mineral, fiber, and phytochemical content) are also extremely valuable to our health. For the glycemic load, the values in this table range from a low of 0 (broccoli, kale, spinach, etc.) to a high of 58 (dried dates). This table uses white bread as the reference for glycemic index. White bread has a glycemic index of 100 when used as the reference food.

Fiber grams are based on the same serving size (generally, a typical serving for that particular food) from which glucose load was determined.

Food	GI	GL	Fiber (g)
BEVERAGES			
milk, whole	38	4	0
milk, skim	46	6	0
chocolate milk (2 percent)	49	12	1.2
Coca-Cola	90	22	0
JUICES			
apple, unsweet	57	17	0.3
carrot juice, fresh	61	14	1
cranberry juice cocktail	97	33	0.3
grapefruit, unsweet	69	12	0.3
orange, unsweet	71	18	0.5
pineapple, unsweet	66	22	0.5
tomato, canned (no added sugar)	54	6	1.1
BREADS			
bagel, white (Lenders)	103	35	1.8
baguette, plain	136	21	1.8
oat-bran bread	63	11	1.4
rye bread	71	8	1.8
white bread	100	14	0.7
100-percent whole-grain bread	73	10	4.5
BREAKFAST CEREALS			
All-Bran (Kellogg's)	54	13	9.7
Bran Chex	83	15	4.9
Cheerios	106	21	2.6
Corn Chex	118	29	0.5
cornflakes	130	33	0.8

Food	GI	GL	Fiber (g)
Corn Pops	114	29	0.4
Cream of Wheat	105	30	3
Crispix	124	30	0.7
Froot Loops	99	25	0.6
Golden Grahams	102	25	0.9
Grape-Nuts	107	22	2.6
oat bran, raw	78	4	1.5
Raisin Bran	87	17	4
Rice Chex	127	32	0.3
Rice Krispies	117	30	0.3
Shredded Wheat	107	21	3
Special K	98	19	0.9
Total	109	24	2.6
GRAINS			
barley, pearl	36	15	5.7
buckwheat	78	22	6
bulgur (cracked wheat), boiled	68	17	7
corn, sweet, cooked	85	20	4
couscous, boiled 5 min.	93	23	2.1
oats, (as porridge)	83	18	4
RICE			
long grain, white unconverted, boiled 15 min.	71	29	0.6
Uncle Ben's parboiled, 20 minutes	107	39	0.6
basmati, white	83	30	0.3
brown rice, steamed	72	22	3

Food	GI	GL	Fiber (g)
DAIRY PRODUCTS			
vanilla ice cream, light (1/2 percent fat)	67	7	0
chocolate ice cream, premium (15 percent fat)	53	6	0.5
milk, whole	38	4	0
milk, skim	46	6	0
vanilla pudding (instant, made with whole milk)	57	8	0
fruit yogurt (low-fat) w/ sugar	47	14	0
fruit yogurt (nonfat) w/ acesulfame K and Splenda	33	6	1
soy milk, reduced-fat	63	11	1
FRUIT			
apple	57	8	4
banana	73	18	3
cherries	32	4	2.8
dates, dried	147	58	4.5
grapefruit, raw	36	4	5
grapes	66	11	1.2
kiwi	68	7	4.1
orange	69	7	3
peach	40	62	.4
pear	54	6	3
pineapple	84	10	1.5

Food	GI	GL	Fiber (g)
plum	34	41	0.8
prunes, pitted	41	14	4.3
raisins	91	28	3
cantaloupe	93	6	1
strawberries	57	1	2.8
watermelon	103	6	0.6
LEGUMES/BEANS			
black-eyed peas	59	18	9.6
garbanzo beans	39	11	6.6
kidney beans (canned)	74	12	14
black beans, soaked overnight, cooked 45 min.	28	7	13.1
lentils, red	36	7	12
pinto beans (dried), boiled	55	14	13
soybeans, green, boiled	25	1	6.3
PREPARED/ CONVENIENCE FOODS			
chicken nuggets	66	10	0.4
fish sticks	54	10	0
french fries, from frozen	107	30	4.5
pizza, cheese, from frozen	86	22	2
pizza, vegetarian (thin crust)	70	17	3
PASTA/NOODLES			
fettuccine, egg noodles	57	25	2
macaroni, boiled 5 min.	64	30	1

Food	GI	GL	Fiber (g)
spaghetti, boiled 5 min.	45	21	3.1
spaghetti, boiled 11 min. (durum wheat semolina)	84	39	3.1
SNACK FOODS			
corn chips	60	15	1.8
fruit bars, strawberry	129	32	0.5
popcorn, plain, cooked in microwave	102	11	3
pretzels, oven-baked	119	22	1
SWEETS			
chocolate (milk)	49	10	1.7
chocolate (white)	63	18	0
Roll-Ups (fruit leather w/ added vitamin C)	142	33	0
jelly beans	112	30	0
M&Ms, peanut	47	8	1
Snickers bar	97	32	1.5
Twix cookie bar	63	24	0.7
NUTS			
cashews	31	4	1.7
peanuts	19	1	4
SUGARS			
honey	78	14	0
sucrose (sugar)	97	10	0
VEGETABLES			
broccoli, steamed	0	0	2.5
kale, cooked	0	0	2
spinach, raw	0	0	2.2

Food	GI	GL	Fiber (g)
zucchini, steamed	0	0	1
lettuce, Romaine	0	0	1
green peas	68	4	4.4
sweet corn, boiled	85	15	2
carrots, boiled and peeled	70	3	3
potato, baked (russet)	121	36	4
sweet potato, baked with skin	69	22	6

Food Step

Step #4: Emphasize heart protective fats and count fat grams for the right balance for your meals and snacks.

You might think food fat is food fat. But there are actually three types of fats in food: saturated fatty acids, polyunsaturated fatty acids, and monounsaturated fatty acids. One of them is better for you than the others. The monounsaturated fats do not seem to promote heart disease, plaque in the arteries, and cancer, as the saturated fats and some of the polyunsaturated fats appear to. It's a no-brainer, then, to start using and eating more monounsaturated fats and definitely less saturated fat.

There are basically two common oils that contain mostly monounsaturated fats: canola oil and olive oil. They each offer additional and different health benefits (you'll find out what those are in the following sections), so I personally use both.

There are certain recipes or foods that I eat that require butter, but only if it is truly the best type of fat for that particular food. Even then, I will use the least amount I can. When I can, I switch to canola oil, olive oil, or canola margarine. In most sautéing circumstances, I can use canola or olive oil. In many baking recipes, such as some cakes, muffins, even pie crust, I can switch to canola oil. If the cookie or cake recipe calls for creaming the shortening or butter with sugar, then usually I can use my favorite margarine. See Chapter 7 for more information.

Canola oil

You may have heard that canola is a "good" fat—that it contains mostly monounsaturated fat. You may have even heard that it is one of the few plant sources of omega-3 fatty acids. But how much would you need to consume to get a potentially beneficial dose of omega-3 fatty acids? I asked researchers at Best Foods, which makes Mazola's Canola Oil, to send me the actual fatty acid breakdown for one tablespoon of canola oil. I was delighted to find that just one tablespoon contained about 1.5 grams omega-3 fatty acids (about the same amount found in 3.5 ounces of cooked salmon). A tablespoon also contains 9 grams of omega-9 fatty acids (such as oleic acid, a monounsaturated fat that may reduce the development of breast carcinomas) and 7 milligrams of mixed tocopherols (a group of antioxidants that includes vitamin E, also known as alpha-tocopherol).

Canola oil has a neutral flavor and can be heated to high temperatures, so I like to use canola oil in baking and frying recipes.

Olive oil

The people in the Mediterranean region have been studied lately because they have surprisingly low rates of heart disease, yet their typical diet can include generous amounts of fat. Their cuisine includes abundant seafood, use of olives and olive oil, fruits, vegetables, beans, and nuts. We now know that all of those foods have health benefits for our body—including olive oil.

Olive oil does not contain omega-3 fatty acids like canola oil does, but the majority of fatty acids in olive oil are still the more beneficial monounsaturated fats; 56 to 83 percent of the fatty acids in olive oil are specifically oleic acid. Canola oil contributes more vitamin E than olive oil, but there is something that olive oil adds to your diet that canola oil doesn't: potentially protective phytochemicals found in olives. I like to use olive oil in my Italian recipes, cold salads, marinades, and vinaigrettes.

Switch to smart fats

Avoiding greasy, high-fat food is a no-brainer, but within that healthier way of eating, we can improve our health even further by making smart fat choices. The smart fats are fish omega-3s, plant omega-3s, and monounsaturated fat.

So what does that mean in terms of cooking fat and baking fat choices? Olive oil is the oil that is highest in monounsaturated fat and it contains some important phytochemicals, but it doesn't contribute any of the plant omega-3s. Canola oil is lowest in saturated fat of the cooking oils and contains an impressive amount of monounsaturated fat and contributes the most plant omega-3s of the vegetable oils.

Monounsaturated fats help reduce the risk of heart disease, especially if they replace saturated or trans fat in the foods we eat. They reduce blood pressure and LDL (bad) cholesterol and may help increase HDL (good) cholesterol. If a diet high in monounsaturated fat is combined with eating fewer carbohydrates, it can also improve insulin sensitivity. Some high monounsaturated fat foods are olive oil, canola oil, peanut oil, hazelnut oil, almonds and almond oil (and some other nuts), and avocados.

Omega-3 fatty acids, especially from fish, may help decrease blood clotting, decrease abnormal heart rhythms, reduce triglycerides, and promote normal blood pressure. Plant omega-3s are also helpful, because your body can convert a small amount of the plant omega-3s into the fish omega-3s. Plus, there is some evidence that plant omega-3s lower heart disease risk as well, through different processes than fish omega-3s. It is also possible that omega-3s help to lower cancer risk; scientists are investigating this area as well. Omega-3s seem to have anti-inflammatory action within body tissue, and some researchers suggest getting more omega-3s to reduce the risk of inflammatory diseases.

Q: Should you count fat grams?

It is helpful for some people with diabetes to count fat grams, because the issue of food fat for most people with type 2 diabetes can be a little tricky. The only way to know what level of fat grams works best for you at what time of day is to count them every now and then. Take a look at your food diary and see what level of fat tends to produce better blood sugars at certain times of day.

Everybody is different, but most people with type 2 diabetes handle carbohydrates better when they are eaten alongside some protein and fat. Fat helps lower the blood glucose response of the other foods it is eaten with. So "some" fat is definitely a good thing—especially if it is one of the more protective type of fats (monounsaturated fat, omega-3, and omega-9 fatty acids). What we are really talking about is a balancing act—pairing your carbohydrate-rich foods (breads, grains, starches, fruits, sweets, etc.) with foods that contribute some protein and fat.

It's a good idea, when you are trying to figure out which foods and food combinations you do best with, to count fat grams along with carbohydrate grams. For many people with type 2 diabetes, meals that are too high in fat (especially saturated and animal fats) can have terrible consequences on after-meal blood sugars. In some people, meals high in animal fats make the body very resistant to insulin. Meals such as sausage and eggs breakfast or your typical pepperoni and sausage pizza can be a blood glucose nightmare.

Cooking with the right fats

If a recipe calls for vegetable oil, just use canola oil. If it calls for vegetable oil and you think the flavor of olive oil would compliment the dish and the oil doesn't need be heated to a high temperature (olive oil starts smoking and breaking down at higher temperatures), then you can even use olive oil instead. But what about the recipes that call for shortening, stick butter, or margarine?

Sometimes I still use butter because that truly is the best fat for that recipe. I just cut it down as far as I can (substituting in other high flavor/high moisture ingredients). But if butter isn't that essential to the recipe, and your original recipe calls for beating the butter, margarine, or shortening in a mixer, usually with sugar then eggs, you can switch to a margarine that lists liquid canola oil as the first ingredient and contains around eight grams of fat per tablespoon. Sometimes you can get away with beating part canola oil and part fat-free cream cheese or sour cream in place of the original fat. If you are just sautéing something in a pan, you can easily switch to canola or olive oil, and you can probably use less than the amount suggested in the original recipe, especially if you are using nonstick pans.

Start collecting recipes that your family likes that call for olive or canola oil. I made up a reduced-fat pie crust recipe that uses canola oil. I now use salad dressings that contain canola or olive oil for my vinaigrette-dependent recipes (such as green salad and pasta salad). These are the kinds of changes you can start making right now.

Food Step

Step #5: Try to keep saturated fat, trans fat, and cholesterol low.

If monounsaturated fat is now "in," then saturated and trans fats are definitely "out." You'd be hard-pressed to find someone who doesn't know that saturated and trans fat are something Americans need to eat less of. High amounts of satu-rated fat are clearly associated with heart disease. More specifi-cally, saturated fat has been shown to raise bad cholesterol (LDL) and triglycerides in the blood, and trans fat lowers HDL (good) cholesterol in addition to raising LDL (bad) cholesterol levels. Obviously, eating less saturated and trans fat is good, solid advice. Giving that advice is easy; following it is the tough part—especially here in the United States. Saturated fat is synonymous with typi-cal American food. It's in hamburgers, french fries, pizza, hot dogs, and apple pie for goodness' sake.

It doesn't matter whether you find your blood sugars improve with a low or moderate fat eating plan, either way, saturated and trans fat and food cholesterol need to be low. Cholesterol should be limited to 200 to 300 milligrams or less a day and saturated fat is supposed to contribute no more than 7 to 10 percent of the total calories (for someone eating 1,800 calories a day, that comes to 14 to 20 grams of saturated fat a day).

The terrible trans fats

Trans fatty acids are unsaturated fatty acids that contain at least one double bond in the "trans" configuration. They occur naturally in low levels in meat and dairy products, but most of the trans fats in the American diet come from trans fats formed during the partial hydrogenation of vegetable oils. This process transforms some of the oil's unsaturated fat into trans fatty acids, which makes them more solid and stable. You'll find trans fats in any cooking or table fats that contain partially hydrogenated fat or oils.

Trans fatty acids are akin to the damaging effects of saturated fat, except trans fats offer a double whammy to your blood lipid profile—in addition to raising your bad cholesterol (LDL) levels, like saturated fat does, trans fats also decrease your good choles-terol (HDL) levels at the same time.

This is one of the reasons why many researchers consider trans fats to be a bigger bad boy than saturated fat. Many researchers suspect that trans fats not only increase your risk for heart disease but may increase the risk for type 2 diabetes, colon cancer, and breast cancer in women.

We should get as little trans fats as possible. Some margarines and shortenings can contain 20 to 40 percent trans fatty acids. There is a new generation of margarines though that are being produced with no or low amounts of trans fat. You can find the amount of trans fat on the nutrition information label now, but keep in mind that if a product has less than 0.5 grams of trans fat per serving, they can put "0" on the label. There are still quite a few products in the supermarket with substantial trans fats, so keep a look out when you are choosing your processed foods.

No more than two grams of trans a day

The American Heart Association advises Americans to consume no more than 2 grams of trans fat per day. That's definitely a best-case scenario. In today's food world, it's easier than you think to eat double or triple the daily 2-gram goal in just one meal, especially if you frequent fast-food chains.

Trans in fast food land

Some of the fast-food chains I researched didn't provide trans fat information in their nutrition information guides (Hardee's, Carl's Jr.), but thankfully many others did include it. This gives us a really good idea of where these trans fats have been hiding, so we can go out of our way to avoid those menu options.

Looking through the following list of the worst trans fat offenders, a few trans fat truths are uncovered:

Trans are often hiding in pastries, pie crust, and biscuits, if the restaurant is using a high trans baking fat. Here are a few examples:

- KFC's Chicken Pot Pie contains a shocking 14 grams of trans fat.
- Arby's Apple or Cherry Turnover contains 6.5 and 6 grams of trans fat, respectively.
- Arby's Cinnamon Twist contains 4 grams trans fat.
- Burger King's Cini-minis contain 4 grams trans fat.
- Chick-fil-A's Hot Buttered Biscuits contain 3 grams of trans and KFC's biscuits contain 3.5 grams of trans fat.

Breaded and fried chicken and seafood can contribute more trans fat than you think. Here are some examples:

- Breaded Clams from Long John Silvers have 2 grams of trans per serving.
- Long John Silver's Crispy Chicken Club Salad contains 6.5 grams of trans fat.
- A piece of battered fish at Long John Silver's is worth 4.5 grams of trans fat.
- An order of McDonald's Breast Strips has 2.5 grams of trans fat.

Trans can be lurking in deep fried potatoes if they are being fried in a cooking fat that contains trans fats. Here are a few examples:

- Small size hash browns from Burger King contains 5 grams of trans fat.
- Burger King's small-sized French Fries contain 3 grams of trans fat.
- A small french fries from McDonalds adds 3.5 grams of trans fat.

Some fast food desserts will add a few grams of trans to the meal total. Here are a few examples:

- McDonald's Baked Apple Pie sounds pretty innocent (it's baked after all) but each one contains 5 grams of trans fat.

- Chick-fil-A's Fudge Nut Brownie contains 2.5 grams of trans fat.

- McDonaldland cookies have 2.5 grams trans fats and one of their sugar cookies will add 2 grams of trans fat.

- Long John Silver's Pecan Pie adds 2 grams of trans fat.

Saturated fat sources

One of the biggest contributors of saturated fat and cholesterol in the American diet is the meat group, which includes beef, processed meats, eggs, poultry, and other meats. In general, if you choose leaner meats, use egg substitute in place of half the eggs (a good rule of thumb), and take the skin off poultry, you will lower the amount of saturated fat and cholesterol.

The dairy group is another saturated fat contributor, so select lower-fat dairy options and you are guaranteed less saturated fat and cholesterol.

Saturated fat is found in other common foods, too, such as butter, ice-cream, lard, bacon, anything made with coconut and palm oil, and vegetables oils that have been "hydrogenated," as is the case with stick margarine and shortening. Many of the packaged foods we buy, such as crackers, cookies, snack foods, frozen fried foods, and pastries contain hydrogenated oils.

Where to cut cholesterol

Plant foods do not contain cholesterol. Where you find high amounts of fat in animals and animal products, generally cholesterol isn't far behind. Food sources highest in cholesterol are egg yolks, organ meats (especially liver), whole-fat dairy products, and higher-fat meats. There are a few fish sources that are a bit higher in cholesterol, such as shrimp, squid, crab, and lobster. But they are low in fat and saturated fat, so don't worry too much about the occasional shrimp cocktail or calamari you enjoy.

Avoiding organ meats is the easy part. Buying skinless chicken is simple, too. And I have personally found it no problem at all to switch to low-fat milk and yogurt, reduced-fat cheese, and fat-free sour cream. The egg substitutes today have come a long way, making it easy to use half real eggs and half egg substitute when cooking. Muffins, cakes, quiches, even omelets still turn out terrific.

Keep in mind that some people show big changes in their serum cholesterol after dietary cholesterol and saturated fat have been increased or decreased, while others show little changes. Blame or thank your genetics. Some people are more sensitive to the cholesterol-raising effects of foods high in saturated fat and cholesterol.

Food
Step

Step #6: Calories do count for many people with type 2 diabetes.

Because we can only lose body fat when the calories we burn are greater than the calories we take in with food, indeed, calories do count. The weight loss can reverse or improve your diabetes and insulin resistance.

Listen to your stomach hunger cues. If you are physically hungry, you should eat. When you are no longer hungry, but comfortable, you should stop eating. But all of this needs to take place while following your carbohydrate budget for each meal. If you are still hungry after eating the amount of food determined by your carbohydrate budget, discuss this with your Certified Diabetes Educator.

Step #7: Eat more fruits and vegetables.

Food Step

Starting your meals and snacks with vegetable soup or green salad is a trick I've learned with my family. Research has confirmed that when vegetables are served as a first course, there is a decrease in the total calories eaten during the meal. If you start your meal by enjoying vegetables, you'll be sure to get some, and they will help fill you up so you won't be as likely to overeat the meat or entrée. Eating at a pizza parlor is a perfect example. While you are waiting for your pizza, relax and enjoy a nice green salad with tomato, kidney beans, and other vegetables (making sure to keep regular dressings to about a tablespoon). You'll find that you won't eat as much pizza. However, if you eat the salad at the same time you eat your pizza, you are less likely to eat the salad.

However, for some people with type 2 diabetes, when fruit is eaten before the meal, it may increase insulin and hunger, thus increasing the risk of overeating at the meal.

There are many health reasons to eat more fruits and vegetables such as high doses of fiber, vitamins and minerals, antioxidants, phytochemicals; and most are naturally low in fat, sugar, and sodium. Often, we just don't get around to eating enough fruits and vegetables. Most people say it is because they aren't as convenient as snack foods and fast food. Others say they simply aren't in the habit. Well, whatever your reason, the time to change is now.

Making fruits and vegetables more habit-forming

I think we would all eat more fruits and vegetables if we just had a mother taking care of us. We need someone to remember to buy the fruits and vegetables, someone to take the time to turn them into beautiful fruit salads or green salads, snack trays, and garnishes or tasty side dishes to our entrées.

Here are some ways to make fruits and vegetables a little more convenient:

- Pack your desk or car with your favorite dried fruits; they will keep for weeks.

- Buy baby carrots and celery sticks and put them out before dinner with a quick dip. (Mix some light or fat-free sour cream with Hidden Valley Ranch dressing powder or onion dip powder to taste.)

- Take time once a week to make a large spinach salad or vegetable-fortified lettuce salad, and just store it (without dressing) in an airtight container. You can have crisp, wonderful salad as a snack or with your lunch or dinner for the next few days.

- Every few days make a point of going to your supermarket and picking out the best tasting and freshest fruits in season. But don't just buy them. Remember you have them, and put them out as a snack for the family. Add a few slices or wedges of fruit to each lunch or dinner plate.

- With a few chops of a knife, you can turn a few pieces of fruit into a beautiful fruit salad. Drizzle lemon, pineapple, or orange juice over the top and toss to coat the fruit with it (the vitamin C helps prevent browning).

- Buy your favorite fruits in the winter—just buy them frozen or canned in juice or light syrup.

- Stock your refrigerator at work and home with your favorite fruit juices (make sure they are 100-percent juice). You can often buy them in individual servings so you can grab them as you are running out the door.

- Make a point to include a vegetable with your lunch.
- Make sure to enjoy vegetables when you eat out at a restaurant or deli.

For a list of fruits and vegetables rich in soluble fiber, refer back to Step #1.

Step #8: Avoid eating large meals.

Food Step   Eating more often, but smaller amounts at a time, is a good idea for some, but can be particularly helpful for some people with type 2 diabetes.

What small meals do for blood sugar levels

Small meals, spaced throughout the day (about every two-and-a-half to three hours,) translate into more stable blood sugars throughout the day. Smaller meals generally result in smaller blood-glucose responses, requiring less insulin and improving blood-glucose control in some people with type 2 diabetes.

It makes sense that the bigger the meal, the larger the number of calories eaten from carbohydrates, fat, and protein, and the higher the blood levels of those nutrients will be after the "large" meal. Large meals also zap you of your after-meal energy. If you've had a large meal, a nap is usually not far behind. But if you eat smaller meals, you will feel more energetic throughout your day. (Smaller, lower-fat meals don't stay in the stomach long; they move quickly to the intestines.) If you feel "light" on your feet, you will be more likely to be physically active, too. The more physically active, the more calories you will burn going about your day.

Other benefits of small meals

If you don't want to eat this way to help your diabetes, then do it for these other great reasons:

- Your brain and body require a constant supply of energy in the blood. Eating smaller, more frequent meals is more likely to keep you blood sugar (and energy) stable, preventing low blood-sugar levels that can trigger headaches, irritability, food cravings, or overeating in susceptible people.

- Eating smaller, more frequent meals is great for appetite control. The more stable blood sugars gained from smaller meals keep us from getting overly hungry, which can lead to overeating or making high-sugar or high-fat food choices.

- One study observed that obesity was less common in people who ate more frequent meals. People who eat smaller, more frequent meals are less likely to overeat at any meal. Larger meals flood your bloodstream with a load of fat, protein, and carbohydrate calories, and your body has to get rid of any extra calories. What does this have to do with being overweight? All extra calories can be converted to body fat for energy storage.

- This is still being investigated, but it is possible that this eating style may help lower serum cholesterol. It stands to reason that by avoiding large meals, you also prevent quick rises of serum triglycerides that typically follow large, particularly fatty meals

- Burn more calories digesting, absorbing, and metabolizing your food just by eating more often. The body burns calories when it digests and absorbs the food we eat. And every time we eat, the digestion process goes into gear. If we eat six small meals instead of two large ones, we start the digestive process three times more often every single day—burning more calories. This metabolism-inspired increase in calories burned can burn around 5 to10 percent of the total calories we eat in a day.

• It's physically more comfortable to eat smaller meals. You aren't weighed down by a large meal in your stomach.

Q: How frequent should the "smaller" meals be?

Experts have not yet determined the ideal eating pattern for people with diabetes, but so far it seems that the closer together the meals are, the better the results. The longer the gap between a previous meal or snack and dinner, for example, the larger the dinner typically ends up being.

If you eat a small breakfast, have a midmorning snack, a light lunch, then an afternoon snack, and a light dinner—it adds up to five small meals for the day. The best advice I can give you, until researchers know more, is to space your meals according to your individual schedule, when you tend to get hungry, and your blood glucose goals.

Fight the urge to eat at night

We burn 70 percent of our calories as fuel during the day, but when do many Americans eat the majority of their calories? During the evening hours. If we're eating small meals throughout the day, eating when we were hungry and stopping when we feel "comfortable," it should be easier to avoid eating large dinners and evening desserts and snacks. Try to keep in mind that what you eat in the evening will be hitting your blood stream pretty much around the time you are getting in your jammies. It isn't as though you are eating to fuel a marathon or anything.

Easier said than done

Our whole society is based on three meals a day, with dinner typically being the largest meal of the day. This is a hard habit to break. If you eat out often, it becomes particularly difficult not to eat a large meal. Restaurants tend to serve large meals—that's all there is to it. It requires extra diligence at restaurants to eat only half your meal and save the rest for later. If you are having spaghetti, you could eat the salad and half your entrée, then have the garlic bread and the rest of your spaghetti later or the next day. I'm not saying it isn't going to be difficult, but it can be done.

A word of caution

Admittedly, for some people this way of eating four or five times a day may not be the best way; these are people who may have a difficult time stopping the eating process once they start. If this describes you, I invite you to visit The Center for Mindful Eating (*www.tcme.org*) for assorted resources to help you be more mindful every time you sit down to enjoy a meal.

Food Step

Step #9: Monitor your blood sugars.

Keeping your blood glucose as near to normal as possible protects your body from diabetic complications further down the line. Measuring your blood sugar levels on a fairly regular basis, then, is a necessary step toward tightly controlling your blood sugar. Measuring your blood sugars will tell you whether you are meeting your treatment goals and whether the agreed-upon treatments (diet, exercise, or pharmacological) are working.

You are hopefully working with a dietitian or diabetes educator who is helping you personalize your eating plan. Logging in your food, blood sugars, medications, and exercise per day shows your dietitian or diabetes educator how your blood sugar is being affected from day to day. Your educator can then work with you on fine-tuning your diabetes care plan by adjusting medications, changing your desired amount of carbohydrate grams, and encouraging activity at certain times.

About one-and-a-half hours after eating you will know whether your blood sugar is within normal limits, high, or low. This is your greatest tool! Use it. Each of us reacts a little differently to each food, combination of foods, and amount of those foods. The only way you can learn your own personal reaction to a particular meal is to test your blood sugar one-and-a-half hours later. Once you begin testing and recording your blood sugar levels, you can look back to your records for clues as to why your readings were what they were. Look for clues in three areas:

1.   Food and diet. (What foods and how much?)
2.   A change in your exercise or activity schedule. (Did you exercise at your usual time for the usual duration?)
3.   Medication. (Did you take the proper amount of medication at the proper time?)

Step #10: Make exercise fun, and do it every day!

When you exercise regularly, you just plain feel better. You burn more calories and you increase your muscle mass, which increases your metabolic rate. And that's just the beginning. Exercising will help decrease blood sugar levels and, possibly, the dose of insulin you need to take. It will decrease blood cholesterol levels and bone loss, while improving your circulation, heart function, and your ability to deal with stress. Obviously, exercise has huge health payoffs.

Make exercise a priority and a habit, please!

4 reasons why many people don't exercise

1. It isn't fun! It isn't exercise, per se, that isn't fun; it's the *type* of exercise that you have been doing that you are not finding fun. Think about all the possible types of exercise and write down which ones you might find the most fun. Also think about what types of exercise you don't like and try to put your finger on why you might not find it fun. This will give you some clues about what your "fun" exercise options might require.

If you dislike the types of exercise that you do alone, then perhaps you would like exercise that is done as a group or team. If you don't think exercising at home is fun, then you should think about exercises—water aerobics, walking with a buddy, country western dance lessons, and so on—that you can do somewhere close to your home.

2. There's just no time! We make time for the things we really *want* to do, don't we? And we make time for the things we really *have* to do, too. If exercising makes us feel better (and we make it fun), then hopefully it will become something we really *want* to do. If exercising helps us control our blood sugar and body weight (and it does!), then it is also something we really *have* to do for our health.

Keep in mind that even fitting 10 minutes of exercise here and there, during our day, can help your body manage diabetes. Walking after a meal or snack (or during a time when your blood sugar tends to be too high) can be particularly helpful for diabetics. The exercise helps move and use the blood sugar in your blood stream. This doesn't have to be jogging or swimming right after a meal, it could be a quick 10-minute jaunt around your office building after lunch, taking the stairs, or walking the dog after dinner.

3. It's boring! You may be someone who needs to plan variety into your exercise program. You might want to join a class (dance, jazzercise, water aerobics, swimming, golf, basketball, or tennis) that meets two or three days a week, then fill in the other days with walks, weight training, cycling, etc. Take lessons for a sport you actually find interesting.

For many of us, exercising at home on a machine is most convenient. If you work out for 30 minutes, then it takes exactly 30 minutes out of your day. I ride my stationary bike while I watch a television movie or program that I'm dying to see. I even fast forward through the commercials if I'm watching a tape. The television keeps my interest while my body is doing the work. You may want to listen to some of your favorite CDs or maybe even an audio book.

4. It's raining, it's pouring! Having several types of exercise options available to you not only adds variety (and minimizes boredom), it gives you an automatic "bad weather" plan. If you have home exercise equipment, use them when the weather is cold or wet. If you have signed up for exercise classes or sports leagues, they are usually indoors, so you know you will at least get some exercise on those days each week.

If you like to walk and you have a walking buddy depending on you, you could very well decide to walk rain or shine. As long as it isn't raining too hard, my walking buddy and I just put our hooded ski jackets on and brave the drops. I find it invigorating! And the warm shower afterwards is truly therapeutic.

Chapter 5

The Recipes You Can't Live Without

This chapter is designed to give you just a sampling of possible recipes to start you on the road to more healthful cooking. Some of the recipes are from scratch, while others make use of the countless convenient products now available. Hopefully you will find a handful that suit you and your family perfectly. I have three cookbooks that might also come in handy: *Food Synergy* (Rodale, March 2008), *Comfort Food Makeovers* (Black Dog & Leventhal, January 2006), and *Fry Light, Fry Right!* (Black Dog & Leventhal, September 2004).

Most of us cook the same recipes over and over again, so I wanted to give you some recipe guidelines to lighten up your own family favorites!

Smart substitutions

Healthy food isn't going to do anyone any good if no one is eating it. That's been my motto for the 15 years that I've been lightening recipes. In other words, even if it's light, it's gotta taste great.

Lightening recipes comes down to basically three things: trimming extra fat and fat-containing ingredients and switching to smart fats when possible, trimming extra sugar and sugar-containing ingredients, and switching to whole grains and adding fiber-rich foods when possible.

The specific keys to successful lightening are:

- Find the ideal fat and sugar threshold for the recipe. How much can you cut calories, fat, and sugar without compromising flavor and texture? See the table on pages 121–123 for more help on this.

- Use the fat substitute that works best in that recipe. See the table for more help on this also.

- Review the functions of each fatty or sweet ingredient before you make changes to your recipe. When fat or sugar serves an irreplaceable function, you'll probably need to keep some of it in, but you can usually cut fat in half and sugar by one-fourth.

- Substitute reduced-fat and reduced-sugar ingredients and products when appropriate. For example, use reduced-fat sharp cheddar cheese instead of regular, use a good-tasting fat-free or light sour cream instead of regular, or use fat-free half-and-half. You can also use reduced-calorie pancake syrup, unsweetened frozen fruit, etc., instead of regular.

- When possible, change to a cooking method that eliminates the need for cooking fat (broiling, roasting, poaching, steaming). But when it is necessary to maintain the character of the food, just use less of it for your oven frying, browning, or sautéing or pan frying.

Ideal fat thresholds and substitutions

Based on two decades of experimentation with the best ways to lighten recipes, I've discovered that there are ideal fat thresholds that you must keep for flavor. If you cut back the fat in a particular recipe, you'll need a "fat replacement" (an extra ingredient you can add to help replace the fat you have taken out).

For example, if you are making brownies and you cut the butter back from 8 tablespoons to 3, you can add 5 tablespoons fat-free sour cream to the batter to make up the difference. You can also use half whole-wheat flour to increase the fiber and you can often reduce the sugar by a third or fourth.

If you are making a spice cake using a cake mix, don't add the 1/2 cup of oil the recipe requires; instead add 1/2 cup of unsweetened applesauce (or some other fat replacement) instead.

Recipe	Fat Threshold	Fat Replacements
Biscuits/Scones	4 Tbs. shortening for every 2 cups flour.	Fat-free cream cheese, nonfat or light sour cream, flavored yogurt.
Cake Mixes	No additional fat is needed because most mixes already contain fat in the mix.	Instead of adding the oil called for on the box, add applesauce, liqueur, fruit juice, flavored yogurt, or nonfat sour cream, depending on the cake.
Brownies	2 1/2 Tbs. canola oil or butter per 4 oz. unsweetened chocolate and about 14 Tbs. flour.	Fat-free sour cream works well, along with espresso or strong coffee.

Recipe	Fat Threshold	Fat Replacements
Homemade cakes and coffee cakes	1/4 to 1/3 cup fat ingredient per cake.	Liqueur for some cakes, light sour cream for chocolate ones; fruit purees and juices work well with carrot, apple, and spice cakes.
Cheese sauce	No butter is needed, so omit the butter if it is called for. The cheese is the vital fatty ingredient; use a reduced-fat cheddar.	Make your thickening paste by mixing the flour with a little bit of milk, then whisk in the remaining milk called for in the recipe.
Cookies	Generally you can only cut the fat by half. If the original recipe calls for 1 cup of butter, try cutting it to 1/2 cup.	Fat-free cream cheese for rich cookies; some fruit purees may work in fruit/drop cookies.
Marinades	1 Tbs. oil per cup of marinade (or none at all).	Fruit juices or beer help to balance the sharpness of the more acid ingredients in a marinade such as vinegar or tomato juice.
Muffins and Nut Bread	2 Tbs. oil for a 12-muffin recipe.	Fat-free sour cream, low-fat flavored yogurts, fruit juice, and fruit purees.

Recipe	Fat Threshold	Fat Replacements
Vinagrette Dressings	1 to 2 Tbs. olive oil per 1/2 cup dressing.	Wine or champagne, fruit juice, fruit purees (raspberry and pear work well).
Cake Mixes	1 tsp. butter per serving of sauce.	Add a little more milk. I like to use whole milk or fat-free half and half for a rich white sauce.

Here are a few more substitution or fat-reduction tips to use when cooking various dishes:

- In mostly egg dishes, you can cut the eggs in half and replace the lost eggs with Egg Beaters egg substitute (1/4 cup substitute per egg).

- Many recipes call for using much more oil or butter in pan frying or sautéing than is really necessary. Using a teaspoon of olive or canola oil, at the most, usually does the trick.

- If you can switch to canola or olive oil instead of using fat or shortening in a recipe, do it! These oils contain better fats (monounsaturated fat and canola oil also contains omega-3s) than the saturated fats in shortening, butter, and stick margarines.

Here are some recipes to get you started!

Three ground flax recipes

Honey Wheat Bread With Flaxseed

I must have experimented with a dozen different bread machine wheat bread recipes and none were great enough for this book—that is, until I found this one! (For 2 pound bread machines.)

Makes 12 slices.

- 1 1/8 cups water
- 2 1/2 cups white bread flour
- 1/2 cup whole wheat flour
- 1 1/2 Tbs. dry milk
- 1 1/2 Tbs. honey
- 1 1/2 tsp. salt
- 2 Tbs. canola oil
- 1/4 cup ground flaxseed
- 3 tsp. active dry yeast (or 2 tsp. fast-rise yeast)

1. Measure your ingredients and one after the other, load them into your bread machine pan. Add them in the order suggested in your machine owner's manual. (Usually you add the liquids first and then the dry ingredients. Make a well in your flour and add the yeast.)

2. Adjust the setting for "wheat bread," and then press "Start." This recipe can also be made with rapid or delayed-time bake cycles.

3. Let the bread cool slightly before removing from the pan. Use a serrated knife to cut into about 12 slices. Enjoy this bread with canola margarine, reduced-fat peanut butter, your favorite preserves, or make your favorite sandwich.

Per serving: 150 calories, 5 g protein, 25 g carbohydrate, 3.8 g fat, 0.5 g saturated fat, 1 mg cholesterol, 2 g fiber, 280 mg sodium. Calories from fat: 19 percent. Omega-3 fatty acid per slice: 0.5 g (1 g per sandwich).

Flaxseed Jam Muffins

Makes 9 regular sized muffins.

- canola cooking spray
- 1/8 cup nonfat or light sour cream
- 1/8 cup canola oil
- 1/2 cup low-fat milk
- 1/4 cup egg substitute (or 1 egg)
- 2 Tbs. light corn syrup
- 1 tsp. vanilla extract
- 2/3 cup unbleached flour
- 2/3 cup whole wheat flour
- 1/3 cup ground flaxseed
- 1/2 cup granulated sugar
- 2 tsp. baking powder
- 1/2 tsp. salt
- 4 Tbs. reduced-sugar jam of your choice

1. Preheat oven to 375 degrees. Coat 9 muffin cups with canola cooking spray.

2. Place sour cream in a glass mixing bowl and warm briefly in the microwave so it will blend easier. Stir in oil and milk, a tablespoon at a time. Stir in egg or egg substitute, corn syrup, and vanilla extract.

3. Blend dry ingredients together (flours, flaxseed, sugar, baking powder, salt) and add all at once to liquid mixture. Stir just enough to moisten.

4. Fill each muffin cup with a level 1/4 cup measure of batter. Spoon about 1 1/2 teaspoons jam in the center of each muffin. Bake about 18 to 20 minutes or until golden brown and muffin tests done.

Per serving: (using reduced-sugar jam) 197 calories, 4.5 g protein, 35.5 g carbohydrate, 5 g fat, .5 g saturated fat, 1 mg cholesterol, 3 g fiber, 260 mg sodium. Calories from fat: 23 percent. Omega-3 fatty acids: 1.5 g.

Flaxseed Maple Scones

If you even barely like the taste of maple, you will find these scones addicting! I even adjusted the recipe for a food processor to make these scones a cinch to make. These scones are loaded with ground flaxseed, so one scone will gives you a day's supply of flaxseed. They freeze well in plastic resealable bags. You can even eat them right out of the freezer!

Makes 8 scones.

Scones:

- 1 1/2 cups all-purpose flour
- 1/3 cup oats
- 1/2 cup ground flaxseed
- 2 Tbs. sugar
- 1/2 tsp. salt
- 1 Tbs. baking powder
- 2 Tbs. maple syrup
- 2 Tbs. canola oil
- 1 egg
- 1/2 cup whole milk (lowfat milk will work too)
- 1/2 tsp. maple extract (3/4 tsp. if you prefer a stronger maple flavor)

- 2/3 cup pecans coarsely chopped (a little smaller than "pecan pieces" but bigger than "finely chopped" pecans)
- canola cooking spray

Maple Glaze:

- 1 1/2 cups powdered sugar
- 1/2 tsp. maple extract
- 5 tsp. water

1. Preheat oven to 425 degrees. Make an 8-inch circle with canola cooking spray on a thick baking sheet.

2. Add flour, oats, flaxseed, sugar, salt, and baking powder to food processor bowl. Pulse to mix and finely grind the oats with the flour.

3. Add maple syrup and canola oil to the flour mixture and pulse to blend well.

4. In a separate small bowl, beat the egg lightly with the milk and 1/2 tsp. maple extract. Pour the milk mixture into the flour mixture in the food processor. Pulse briefly to make a dough.

5. Place dough on well-floured surface. Sprinkle pecans over the top and knead lightly four times to evenly distribute the pecans. Pat dough into a 7 1/2-inch circle. Cut into 8 wedges. Place wedges in a circle on prepared baking sheet. Bake in center of oven for about 13–15 minutes (top will be lightly browned).

6. While scones are baking, add glaze ingredients to a small bowl and stir well until smooth. Remove scones from oven to wire rack and let cool about three to five minutes. Spread glaze generously over each scone. Once glaze has dried (about 15 minutes) the scones can be served! They keep well overnight in a resealable plastic bag.

Per serving: 330 calories, 6 g protein, 51 g carbohydrate, 12 g fat, 4 g fiber, 38 mg cholesterol, 370 mg sodium. Calories from fat: 33 percent. Omega-3 fatty acids: 1.3 g.

Note: Because the fat grams mainly come from the pecans and the canola oil, most of the fat is the preferred monounsaturated fat!

Best bean recipes

High Legume Fried Rice

Makes 4 servings.

- 3 Tbs. canola oil
- 1/4 cup green onions, sliced, firmly packed
- 3/4 cup frozen green peas
- 3/4 cup shelled edamame (If using frozen pods, follow the directions on the bag to finish cooking, then remove the soy beans from the pods before measuring).
- 1/2 cup diced lean ham (optional)
- 4 cups cooked steamed brown rice
- 1 egg beaten with 1/4 cup egg substitute
- 1/2 tsp. salt
- 1 to 2 Tbs. light or regular soy sauce

1. Heat oil in wok or large nonstick saucepan to very hot. Add green onion and let sit for one minute.

2. Add green peas, soy beans, ham, and rice. Let stand for a minute.

3. Push away the mixture toward the edges of the pan, leaving the middle of the pan open, and pour in the egg mixture.

4. Let sit for about 20 seconds, then begin to stir the eggs for another 20 seconds.

5. Stir fry the entire mixture together for a couple of minutes, sprinkling salt and soy sauce over the top. Add more soy sauce at table if desired.

Per serving: (with 2 Tbs. light soy sauce) 412 calories, 14.5 g protein, 64 g carbohydrate, 10 g fat, 1.5 g saturated fat, 53 mg cholesterol, 9 g fiber, 590 mg sodium. Calories from fat: 28 percent.

The 3-Minute Burrito

Makes 1 burrito.

- 1/2 cup cooked or canned pinto beans or pinquitos (small brown beans), drained and rinsed
- 1 Tbs. chopped fresh cilantro (optional)
- 2 Tbs. light or fat-free sour cream
- 1 green onion, chopped
- 1/8 cup chunky salsa (mild or hot, depending on preference)
- 1 burrito-size flour tortilla
- 1 1/2 ounces reduced-fat Monterey jack or sharp cheddar cheese, grated (about a heaping 1/3 cup)

1. In small bowl, toss beans, cilantro, sour cream, green onion, and salsa together.

2. Heat tortilla in microwave on a double thickness of paper towel for about 1 minute or until soft.

3. Sprinkle cheese evenly over the tortilla.

4. Spread bean mixture in center of tortilla. Fold bottom and top ends of tortilla in and roll up into a burrito.

5. Microwave 1 more minute or until burrito is heated through.

Per serving: 430 calories, 23.5 g protein, 53.5 g carbohydrate, 14.5 g fat, 7 grams saturated fat, 26 mg cholesterol, 6 g fiber, 480 mg sodium. Calories from fat: 30 percent.

Breakfast ideas

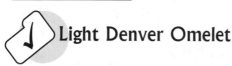

Light Denver Omelet

I know this looks like it takes a bit of time, what with whipping egg whites and everything, but once you know what you're doing, you can turn this out in 10 minutes. If you don't want to whip the egg whites, just beat them into the rest of the egg mixture (it won't be as fluffy, but it still tastes great).

Makes 2 servings.

- canola cooking spray
- 1 cup sliced fresh mushrooms (or other vegetable)
- 1 medium green pepper, chopped
- 4 green onions, sliced diagonally
- 1/4 tsp. dried basil
- 1/2 cup chicken broth (water can also be used)
- 3 ounces (1/2 cup slightly heaping) lean ham, cut into 2-inch long strips
- 1/2 cup cherry tomatoes, halved (or other tomatoes)
- 1/2 cup egg substitute
- 2 eggs, separated

1. Coat a medium nonstick frying pan with canola cooking spray, and heat over medium heat. Add mushrooms, green pepper, green onions, and basil. Sauté

about 30 seconds, then pour in the chicken broth and cook, stirring frequently, until vegetables are tender. Stir in ham and cherry tomatoes and cook about a minute to heat through.

2. Blend egg substitute and egg yolks in medium-sized bowl and set aside. With mixer, beat egg whites until stiff. Carefully fold egg whites into egg-yolk mixture.

3. Coat a nonstick omelet pan or small nonstick frying pan with canola cooking spray (or use 1/2 tsp. canola oil or canola margarine), and heat over medium-low heat. Spread half of egg mixture in pan. Heat until top looks firm (about two minutes). If your pan cooks hotter than normal (as some nonstick pans do), cook over low heat. Flip omelet over to lightly brown other side (about one minute).

4. Fill with half of the vegetable-ham filling, and fold as desired. Remove to serving plate. Repeat with remaining egg mixture to make a second fluffy omelet.

Per serving: 190 calories, 9 g carbohydrate, 22 g protein, 7 g fat, 2 g saturated fat, 229 mg cholesterol, 2 g fiber, 690 mg sodium. Calories from fat: 35 percent.

 ## Egg Muffin Sandwich Lite

Makes 2 sandwiches.

- 2 whole grain English muffins, toasted
- 1 egg
- 1/4 cup egg substitute
- 2 slices Canadian bacon (or thick slices lean ham)
- 1 6.5-oz empty tuna can (or similar), washed, labels removed

- freshly ground pepper
- 2 slices 1/3 low-fat American cheese slices (or similar)
- canola cooking spray

1. Coat half of a 9-inch nonstick frying pan with canola cooking spray, and heat over medium heat.
2. In small bowl, beat the egg with egg substitute; set aside.
3. Place Canadian bacon in the pan over the spray coated area. Spray inside of tuna can with canola cooking spray, and set can on the other side of the pan to start heating. When bottom side of the bacon is light brown, flip over to the other side and cook until light brown. Remove slices from pan and set aside.
4. Pour half of egg mixture (1/4 cup) into tuna can. Sprinkle with freshly ground pepper to taste. When the surface of egg begins to firm, cut around the inside of the can with a butter knife to free the edges. Turn the egg over with a cake fork, and cook one minute more.
5. Remove egg from can.
6. Coat can with canola cooking spray. Repeat with remaining egg.
7. To assemble, layer English muffin bottom with a slice of cheese, then egg, a piece of Canadian bacon, and the English muffin top. To reheat, microwave each sandwich for 20 seconds on high.

Per serving: 287 calories, 21.5 g protein, 30.5 g carbohydrate, 9 g fat, 3.8 g saturated fat, 130 mg cholesterol, 5 g fiber, 1,100 mg sodium. Calories from fat: 28 percent.

Sun-Dried Tomato Pesto Bagel Spread

Makes spread for about 3 bagels.

- 1/2 cup light or Neufchâtel cream cheese
- 1 clove garlic, minced or pressed
- 1 Tbs. basil leaves, fresh and chopped
- 1 Tbs. julienne-style sun-dried tomatoes from bag, soaked in warm water until tender, then drained
- 2 Tbs. pine nuts, pecans, or walnuts

Add all ingredients to small food processor and process until well blended. Spread on bagels.

Per serving: (with whole grain bagel) 300 calories, 40 g carbohydrate, 14 g protein, 9 g fat, 4.5 g saturated fat, 20 mg cholesterol, 8 g fiber, 205 mg sodium. Calories from fat: 27 percent.

 ## The Lox-ness Monster Bagel Spread

Makes about 1/2 cup of spread (enough for about 4 bagels).

- 1/2 cup light cream cheese
- 2 ounces lox, finely chopped
- 1 green onion, finely chopped
- pinch of fresh or dried dill (optional)
- pinch of capers (optional)

Blend all ingredients in food processor until well mixed. You should still be able to see some small pieces of lox. Spread on bagels.

Per serving: (with whole-wheat bagel) 270 calories, 13 g protein, 38.5 g carbohydrate, 7 g fat, 3.5 g saturated fat, 18 mg cholesterol, 4 g fiber, 560 mg sodium. Calories from fat: 23 percent.

Apple Lover's Oatmeal

Makes 1 serving.

- 1 packet instant oatmeal, plain. (If you use flavored, sweetened instant oatmeal, such as "maple & brown sugar" then don't add the brown sugar.)
- 1 individual serving applesauce (3.9 oz), unsweetened (1/3 cup)
- 1 Tbs. brown sugar
- 1/4 tsp. ground cinnamon
- 1/2 cup lowfat milk (or similar—soy milk or almond milk can also be used)

In a large microwave-safe soup bowl, blend all ingredients together. Microwave on high for 1 1/2 minutes. Stir, then microwave for another 1 1/2 minutes. Serve hot.

Per serving: 180 calories, 5.5 g protein, 35 g carbohydrate, 2 grams fat, .8 g saturated fat, 5 mg cholesterol, 2.5 g fiber, 140 mg sodium. Calories from fat: 10 percent.

Note: To make a more balanced breakfast, enjoy this oatmeal with a strip or two of Louis Rich turkey bacon.

Scrumptious side dishes

 ## Monounsaturated Side Salad

This salad is not just rich in monounsaturated fats—it's rich in fiber.

Makes 4 servings.

- 1/2 avocado, cut into bite-size pieces
- 1/2 cucumber, sliced

- 1 cup chopped tomatoes or cherry tomatoes cut in half
- 1 cup kidney beans (or 1/2 cup kidney beans and 1/2 cup garbanzo), drained and rinsed
- 6 Tbs. Wish-Bone Olive Oil Vinaigrette (or other dressing that uses olive oil or canola oil)
- 4 to 6 cups read-to-serve salad greens of your choice

1. Place avocado, cucumber, tomatoes, and beans into a serving bowl. Toss with dressing; set aside in refrigerator until needed.
2. Right before mealtime, toss vegetable mixture with lettuce.

Per serving: 155 calories, 6 g protein, 19 g carbohydrate, 7 g fat, 0.7 g saturated fat, 0 mg cholesterol, 7 g fiber, 460 mg sodium. Calories from fat: 43 percent.

 Easy 3-Bean Salad

Makes 4 servings.

- 1 8.75-ounce can kidney beans, drained and rinsed (about 1 cup)
- 1 8.75-ounce can garbanzo beans, drained and rinsed (about 1 cup)
- 1 8.75-ounce can green or yellow wax beans, drained and rinsed (about 1 cup)
- 1/4 cup finely diced yellow or white onion
- 4 Tbs. bottled vinaigrette (that uses olive oil or canola oil)

Add all ingredients to serving bowl. Toss well. This will store covered in the refrigerator for several days.

Per serving: 160 calories, 7 g protein, 27.5 g carbohydrate, 3 g fat, 0 g saturated fat, 0 mg cholesterol, 7 g fiber, 635 mg sodium. Calories from fat: 17 percent.

Quick snacks and pick-me-ups

 Spicy Hummus With Crudités and Crackers

This is a variation on the really tasty middle Eastern dip/spread. You may have to search a bit to find tahini, although it is available in many supermarkets on the East and West Coasts.

Makes about 3 cups of dip.

- 1 15.5-oz. cans 50 percent less sodium garbanzo beans
- 3 cloves garlic, minced or pressed
- 1/3 cup tahini (sesame seed paste)
- 1/4 cup lemon juice
- 3 Tbs. light or fat-free sour cream
- 2 Tbs. light cream cheese
- 1/4 tsp. seasoning salt (optional)
- 1/4 tsp. ground cumin
- 1/4 tsp. paprika
- 2 Tbs. finely chopped fresh parsley (optional)
- Crudités: choose crisp vegetables such as red bell pepper, carrots, celery, cauliflower, broccoli, green beans, etc.
- Crackers: choose from many reduced-fat crackers on the market.

1. Drain garbanzo beans and rinse well. (Reserve some of the liquid to add back if you need it to make a thinner dip.)

2. Place beans, garlic, tahini, lemon juice, sour cream, cream cheese, seasoning salt, cumin, paprika, and parsley in food processor. Blend until somewhat smooth. Add more lemon juice or garbanzo liquid to taste. Use immediately or cover and refrigerate (will keep for several days). Serve with vegetables and crackers.

Per serving: (1/3 cup dip) 100 calories, 1 g protein, 9 g carbohydrate, 5.5 g fat, 1 g saturated fat, 1 mg cholesterol, 3 g fiber, 120 mg sodium. Calories from fat: 50 percent.

When each serving is eaten with a cup of suggested vegetables, the fiber increases to about 6 grams a serving.

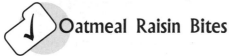Oatmeal Raisin Bites

You can make a batch of these babies then pop them in the freezer in a resealable plastic bag. Take out a cookie whenever you need one. They thaw quickly in the microwave or at room temperature.

Makes 32 large cookies.

- 6 Tbs. canola margarine or butter, softened
- 6 Tbs. fat-free or light cream cheese
- 1 cup packed brown sugar
- 1/2 cup granulated sugar
- 1/4 cup low-fat buttermilk
- 1/4 cup egg substitute
- 2 Tbs. maple syrup
- 2 Tbs. vanilla extract
- 1 cup whole wheat flour (unbleached flour can be used)
- 1/2 tsp. baking soda
- 1 1/2 tsp. ground cinnamon
- 1/4 tsp. salt

- 2 cups quick or old fashioned oats
- 1 cup raisins
- 1/2 cup chopped walnuts (optional)

1. Preheat oven to 350 degrees. Coat two cookie sheets with canola cooking spray. In a large bowl, beat the butter with cream cheese. Beat in the sugars, buttermilk, egg substitute, maple syrup, and vanilla until light and fluffy.
2. Combine the flour, baking soda, cinnamon, and salt; beat into the butter mixture.
3. Stir in the oats, raisins, and nuts if desired, mixing well.
4. Use a cookie scoop (or drop by rounded tablespoonfuls) to form cookies and place 2 inches apart on the prepared cookie sheets. For flatter (rather than rounded) cookies, press each cookie mound down lightly with a spoon, spatula, or your fingers.
5. Bake one cookie sheet at a time, in the upper third of oven for about 10 minutes, or until lightly browned. Remove the cookies to wire racks to cool completely. Store in an airtight container.

Per serving: 120 calories, 2 g protein, 22 g carbohydrate, 3 g fat, .4 g saturated fat, 5 mg cholesterol, 2 g fiber, 36 mg sodium. Calories from fat: 22 percent.

Quick Omega-3 Entrées

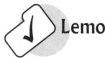 **Lemon Dijon Salmon**

Makes 2 servings.

- 2 salmon steaks (about 6 ounces each)
- 1 Tbs. Dijon mustard

- Garlic salt (about 1/2 tsp.)
- Freshly ground pepper
- 1/2 onion, thinly sliced
- 1/2 lemon
- 2 to 3 tsp. capers

1. Preheat oven to 400 degrees. Line a 9-inch pie plate with a large sheet of foil (enough so it can be wrapped back over the fish and sealed) and spray foil generously with canola cooking spray. Lay salmon steaks in prepared pan.

2. Spread fish steaks evenly with Dijon mustard.

3. Sprinkle fish steaks with garlic salt and ground pepper to your liking.

4. Lay thinly sliced onion over the top.

5. Squeeze 1/2 lemon over the top of the salmon and sprinkle capers over the top.

6. Wrap edges of foil over the top of fish and seal edges together. Bake about 15 minutes. Open foil and let bake about 5 minutes more or until salmon is cooked throughout.

7. Serve with steamed brown rice or cooked pasta and some vegetables.

Per serving: 231 calories, 30 g protein, 5 g carbohydrate, 10 g fat, 1.5 g saturated fat, 80 mg cholesterol, 1 g fiber, 678 mg sodium. Calories from fat: 39 percent.

Per serving: (when each serving is served with 3/4 cup steamed brown rice and a cup of broccoli) 475 calories, 38.5 g protein, 56 g carbohydrate, 11 g fat, 1.7 g saturated fat, 80 mg cholesterol, 8 g fiber, 720 mg sodium. Calories from fat: 21 percent. Omega 3 fatty acids: 1.5 g.

Simple Salmon Pasta Salad

This is one of my favorite salads. When I cook grilled salmon, I make extra on purpose so I can make this salad the next day with the leftovers.

Makes about 2 entrée servings.

Salmon:

- 2 cups whole wheat blend bow tie or rotelle pasta, cooked al dente
- 1 cup salmon flakes (freshly cooked or grilled salmon fillets or steaks, broken into flakes with fork, with no bones or skin)
- 1 cup crisp-tender asparagus pieces, steamed or microwaved
- 3 green onions, finely chopped

Dressing:

- 1 Tbs. canola mayo or light mayonnaise
- 2 Tbs. fat-free or light sour cream
- 1 Tbs. lemon juice
- 1 1/2 tsp. Dijon or prepared mustard
- 1/2 tsp. dill weed
- Black pepper to taste

1. Place pasta, salmon, asparagus, and green onions in serving bowl.
2. Blend dressing ingredients until smooth. Add to pasta salad ingredients and stir to mix.

Per serving: 339 calories, 18 g protein, 45 g carbohydrate, 9.5 g fat, 1.5 g saturated fat, 29 mg cholesterol, 7 g fiber, 122 mg sodium. Calories from fat: 26 percent. Omega-3 fatty acid per serving: 1 g.

Easy Omega-3 Fatty Acid Tuna Sandwich

- 6 1/2 ounces albacore tuna, canned in spring water, drained
- 1 Tbs. sweet or dill pickle relish (optional)
- 1/4 tsp. salt (optional)
- 1 Tbs. canola mayo or light mayonnaise
- 1/2 Tbs. minced onion
- 1/4 cup minced celery
- 1 Tbs. light or fat-free sour cream
- pepper to taste
- 2 slices whole wheat or whole grain bread (toasted if desired)
- lettuce leaves and tomato slices

1. Combine tuna, relish, salt, mayo, sour cream, onion, and celery in small bowl; mix well. Add pepper to taste.
2. Spread mixture on slices of bread to make a sandwich. Add lettuce leaves and tomato slices.

Per serving: 320 calories, 27 g protein, 34 g carbohydrate, 8.5 g fat, 1.4 g saturated fat, 27 mg cholesterol, 4.5 g fiber, 676 mg sodium. Calories from fat: 25 percent. Omega-3 fatty acids: about 0.5g from tuna and about 0.5 from the canola mayonnaise.

Other quick entrées

Oat Bran Meat Loaf

This meat loaf tastes so much better than it sounds. Each serving contributes 5 grams of mostly soluble fiber to the meal too!

Makes 5 servings

- 1 1/4 cup canned chickpeas (garbanzo beans), drained and rinsed
- 1/2 cup oat bran
- 1/2 tsp. black pepper
- 1/2 tsp. salt (optional)
- 2 cloves garlic, minced or pressed, or 1/2 teaspoon garlic powder
- 1 Tbs. Worcestershire sauce
- 2 Tbs. Heinz chili sauce
- 1 Tbs. prepared mustard
- 1 lb. ground sirloin (about 9 percent fat) or extra lean ground beef
- 1 cup grated, reduced-fat, sharp cheddar cheese (optional)
- 1 small onion, finely chopped
- canola cooking spray
- 1 cup tomato sauce

1. Preheat oven to 350 degrees. Coat a 9-by-5-inch loaf pan with canola cooking spray.
2. Add ingredients up to and including mustard to mixer or food processor. You can also mash with pastry blender or potato masher.
3. Process until well mixed (there will still be some lumps).
4. If using a mixer, add beef, cheese, and onion to bean mixture and mix until well blended. If using a food processor, blend bean mixture with beef, cheese, and onion with hands (or use a spoon) in a large mixing bowl.
5. Add mixture to pan and form into a loaf.

6. Bake 30 minutes. Pour tomato sauce over the top and bake 15 minutes longer.

Per serving: 286 calories, 24.5 g protein, 28.5 g carbohydrate, 10 g fat, 3.5 g saturated fat, 33 mg cholesterol, 5 g fiber, 700 mg sodium. Calories from fat: 29 percent.

Light Club Sandwich

Makes 1 sandwich.

- 2 slices Louis Rich turkey bacon
- 2 slices whole wheat bread
- 1 tsp. canola mayonnaise or light mayo blended with 1 tsp. of light or fat-free sour cream
- 2 lettuce leaves
- 1 large slice turkey breast (about 2 ounces)
- Pepper to taste
- 1/2 large tomato, sliced

1. Cook bacon in nonstick frying pan, over low heat, until crisp.

2. Spread one side of each bread slice lightly with mayonnaise mixture. Arrange lettuce leaf on one slice; top with one slice of turkey; sprinkle with pepper, then cover with another bread slice, mayonnaise side up. Top with another leaf of lettuce, tomato slices, bacon slices, and remaining bread slice, mayonnaise side down.

3. Cut sandwich diagonally into fourths; secure each quarter with decorated toothpicks if desired.

Per serving: 350 calories, 19 g protein, 38 g carbohydrate, 12.5 g fat, 2.7 g saturated fat, 49 mg cholesterol, 5.5 g fiber, 1,400 mg sodium. Calories from fat: 32 percent.

Chapter 6
Navigating the Supermarket

It's easy to get confused while shopping in the trenches (a.k.a. your typical grocery store). Each product label your eye catches inevitably hits you with countless advertising slogans and nutrition terms. Just remember the bottom line is that all these companies are basically trying to sell you something; they all want a piece of your food budget. The package might boast "sugar-free" or "fat-free," but it's the nutrition information label that's going to tell you whether that product has just as many grams of carbohydrate or just as many calories as the regular products.

It's also the nutrition information label that is going to confess what the company considers the serving size to be. The serving size of many individual or small frozen pizzas is 1/3 of the "small" pizza. There are some reduced-fat ice cream bars out there that, when you check the label, still contain more than 13 grams of fat per serving. The moral of this story is to read your labels. You'll get the information you need for counting and calculating from the nutrition information label—check the portion size, the grams of fat, carbohydrates, and calories when shopping for and comparing food products.

The second lesson is a bit more difficult to master. Some of us may be using these fat-free products as an excuse to overeat. I don't think we are entirely to blame here. If these products aren't as satisfying, we're probably more likely to keep on eating and eating in the hope of reaching some level of satisfaction. Also, some of the advertising has basically encouraged us to eat as much as we want— after all, it's fat-free! So select light and fat-free products that you truly like—that taste satisfying to you—that you can eat in modest serving sizes. Otherwise, they aren't going to do a hill of beans for your health and enjoyment.

Avoiding the land mines

Have you ever noticed that the nutrition facts information on the label of a baking mix or cake mix is listed in two columns? It is usually gives to sets of information, one for *Mix* and one for *Baked* (or *As Prepared*). Normally they will give you two amounts of fat grams; one from the mix and one for the total amount of fat per serving after it's prepared. This is important information, because many of these mixes call for 1/3 cup of oil, three eggs, or a stick of butter.

Several companies have started giving only the grams of fat in the mix. If you look real closely, which is what I get paid to do, you'll see a tiny asterisk next to the grams of fat. Then you look down at the very bottom of the label and in small print it reads something like this: "Amount in mix."

They do give you the percent daily value for grams of fat "as prepared," but let's face it, what does that really mean to most people? Most people just quickly scan the label until they see grams of fat. I can just picture people thinking, "Oh, goody, 4 grams of fat!" When in reality, if they follow the directions on the box, a serving has something more like 9 or 13 grams of fat per serving.

Just so you know what to watch out for, here is an example:

A serving of Pillsbury Thick 'n Fudgy Cheesecake Swirl Deluxe Brownie Mix contains 4.5 grams of fat. When you follow the directions on the box, adding 1/4 cup oil and two eggs to the mix, the grams of fat per serving increases to 9 grams of fat. But you won't see 9 grams anywhere on the label. If you look really hard you'll find 14 percent daily value for fat in the "prepared" column. You have to do a little math to get to 9 from the 14 percent daily value given on the label.

It's all in a name

We've come to rely on certain brands with diet-sounding names to steer us toward the better choices where our waistlines and diabetes are concerned. Weight Watchers, Lean Cuisine, and Slim Fast, for example, are all music to the ears. But don't let those seductive names fool you. Some of these products are just as high in calories, fat, and carbohydrate grams as the overtly "sinful" products farther down the aisle.

In many cases, what they are selling you is portion control and a pretty name (for a handsome price). Keep your eyes open and read the label!

Fat-free, but full of calories

Here's a news flash—just because a product is fat-free doesn't mean it is calorie-free or that you can eat the whole box in one sitting. In fact, many of these fat-free products have just as many calories as the full-fat versions. How can that be? In a word—*sugar*. Sugar, whether it comes from honey, corn syrup, brown sugar, or high fructose corn syrup, can add moisture and help tenderize bakery products. When added to foods such as ice cream, it adds flavor and structure. So I'm not surprised that manufacturers have turned to sugar for assistance while developing reduced-fat and fat-free products.

The majority of the fat-free and lower-fat products on the supermarket shelves only offer us average savings of 10 or 20 calories per serving. Does this mean we shouldn't buy any of these products? No—this means to truly benefit from these lower-fat or fat-free products, we need to watch our serving size and keep track of the grams of carbohydrates we are taking in.

Taking a tour of your supermarket

Next time you walk around your supermarket, aisle by aisle, look for smarter foods and products that offer:

- Lower-carbohydrate, lower-sugar, and reduced-calorie products that might come in handy when you are trying to balance a meal or snack.
- Good, easy sources of soluble fiber (and fiber in general).
- Products and foods that feature the smart fats—omega-3 fatty acids and monounsaturated fats.
- Whole-grain products that would contribute fiber and other nutrients, and also possibly have a positive effect on our blood sugars.

I've included some product information for some of the food/product categories that I thought might help you the most.

Choosing a healthy breakfast cereal

The cereal aisle is a long one, full of contradictions. You'll find cereals made with refined grains with nearly no fiber, and cereals made with whole grains and bran boasting 7 grams or more of fiber. There are cereals with so much sugar they seem more like boxes of little cookies. And, luckily, there are cereals with sugar listed far down on the ingredient list.

Choosing a healthy breakfast cereal is mainly about getting some whole grains. There's no excuse not to get at least one serving of whole grains if you eat cereal for breakfast. And it's well worth the effort; recent research suggests those who eat more whole grains are at lower risk of diabetes and heart disease.

Cereals made with refined grains have generally not been linked to health benefits, such as a lower risk of death from heart disease, as whole-grain breakfast cereals have. Refined-grain cereals do not lower the risk of gaining weight or having a higher BMI (body mass index), but whole grain–rich cereals do.

Q: Taste or nutrition?

Of course, one person's perfect whole-grain cereal with less sugar is another person's bowl of sawdust. If you like breakfast cereals that come in lots of colors and artificial flavors, then, yes, you probably do have to choose between taste and nutrition. But if you like a cereal with natural flavors from toasted whole grains, and maybe some nuts and dried fruit, you'll have many healthful cereals to choose from.

And, yes, dried fruits do add nutrition to your cereal. A quarter of a cup of raisins, for example, has about 1.5 grams of fiber plus 4 percent of the recommended daily value for vitamin E and about 6 percent each of the daily value for vitamins B-1, B-6, and iron, magnesium, and selenium. But when you look on the nutrition facts label for Raisin Bran, for example, you might be shocked to see there are 19 grams of sugar in a 1-cup serving. What's going on is that any sugars—even those from natural sources such as dried fruit—are counted in the sugar grams listed on the label.

Focus on the grams of carbohydrate per serving of the cereal, because this is going to be what you count in your carbohydrate budget for that meal.

Q: Does bran matter?

Bran's biggest benefit is boosting the grams of fiber per serving. This makes the cereal seem more filling, both in the short run and a couple of hours. This staying power may have something to do with the lower glycemic index of bran cereals. One study noted that the glycemic index of corn flakes was more than twice that of bran cereal.

Other recent research found that adding bran to the diet reduced the risk of weight gain in men aged 40–75. Another study, in women aged 38–63, reported that as intake of fiber and whole-grain foods went up, the rate of weight gain tended to decrease. Eating refined grains had the opposite effect. As the intake of refined-grain foods increased, so did weight gain.

Q: How much sugar?

Does the ingredients list for your cereal look a lot like that on, say, a box of cookies? One ounce of Mini Oreo cookies has 11 grams of sugar and 130 calories (34 percent of its calories come from sugar). And sugar is the second ingredient listed (enriched flour is first). Lots of cereals have ingredient lists that look similar—such as Cookie Crisp cereal, with 44 percent of calories from sugar.

The U.S. Government's Dietary Reference Intakes recommend that added sugars not exceed 25 percent of total calories (to ensure sufficient intake of micronutrients). And while there isn't a specific guideline for cereal, it makes sense to aim for a cereal that gets 25 percent or less of its calories from sugar. (If the cereal contains dried fruit, this could be a pinch higher.)

To calculate the percentage of calories from sugar in your cereal:

1. Multiply the grams of sugar per serving by four (there are four calories per gram of sugar).
2. Divide this number (calories from sugar) by the total number of calories per serving.
3. Multiply this number by 100 to get the percentage of calories from sugar.

While you can find plenty of cereals with 5 grams of fiber per serving or more, some of them go a little bit over the "25 percent of calories from sugar" guideline. But if the percentage of sugar calories is still below 30 percent, the first ingredient is a whole grain, and the cereal tastes good, it may still be a good choice overall. Here are two examples.

Kellogg's Frosted Mini-Wheats Strawberry Delight has 5 grams of fiber and 12 grams of sugar per serving (about 27 percent of calories from sugar). The first three ingredients are whole-grain wheat, sugar, and strawberry-flavored crunchlets (sugar, corn cereal, corn syrup are the first three ingredients for these). A pleasant surprise: the strawberry coating creates a strawberry-flavored milk when you pour milk in your cereal.

Kashi GoLean Crunch has 8 grams of fiber and 13 grams of sugar per serving (27 percent of calories from sugar). The first three ingredients are Kashi Seven Whole Grains & Sesame Cereal (whole oats, long grain brown rice, rye, hard red winter wheat, triticale, buckwheat, barley, sesame seeds); textured soy protein concentrate; and evaporated cane juice. This is basically a Kashi-fied version of granola, and 3 grams of the 8 grams of fiber are from soluble fiber (thanks to the oats and barley).

Eight good-tasting picks

After some taste testing and input from acquaintances, I came up with eight picks for the best-tasting healthful breakfast cereals. The cereals on my list had to have a whole grain as the first ingredient and 5 grams of fiber per serving. Sugar had to be around

25 percent of calories from sugar or less, unless dried fruit was among the top three ingredients. I also tried to choose cereals that are easily found in the supermarket.

- **Post Grape-Nuts Trail Mix Crunch:** 5 grams fiber, and 22 percent of calories from sugar. The first three ingredients are whole grain wheat, malted barley, and sugar, followed by raisins and wheat bran.

- **Fiber One Bran Cereal:** 14 grams fiber, 0 percent of calories from sugar. First three ingredients are whole-grain wheat bran, corn bran, and cornstarch. This cereal only appeals to some people. I would suggest enhancing the flavor with cinnamon, fresh or dried fruit, and/or roasted nuts.

- **Fiber One Honey Clusters:** 13 grams fiber, 15 percent of calories from sugar. The first three ingredients are whole-grain wheat, corn bran, and wheat bran.

- **Quaker Oatmeal Squares:** 5 grams fiber, 19 percent of calories from sugar. The first three ingredients are whole oat flour, whole-wheat flour, and brown sugar.

- **Shredded Wheat:** 6 grams fiber, 0 percent of calories from sugar (for a generic brand). The only ingredient is 100 percent whole grain cereal. I enjoy this with added fresh or dried fruit and nuts. If you opt for the frosted variety, it has 6 grams fiber and gets 23 percent of its calories from sugar.

- **Frosted Mini Wheats:** 6 grams fiber, 24 percent of calories from sugar. The first three ingredients are whole-grain wheat, sugar, and high-fructose corn syrup.

- **Kellogg's Raisin Bran:** 7 grams fiber, 40 percent of calories from sugar. The first three ingredients are whole wheat, raisins, and wheat bran. Sugar is listed fourth in the ingredient list, but many of the calories from sugar come from the raisins.

- **Kashi Heart to Heart Honey Toasted Oat Cereal:** 5 grams fiber, 18 percent of calories from sugar. The first three ingredients are whole oat flour, oat bran, and evaporated cane juice. This is a higher-fiber alternative to Cheerios. I think they taste better, too. But that may be because there is more sweetener added (the evaporated cane juice).

Diabetic-friendly frozen entrées

Frozen entrees come in handy in many situations—as a quick lunch during the workweek and as an easy dinner if you live alone or with one other person.

The problem with frozen entrées is that the ones that are lower in fat are almost always too low in calories and carbohydrate, and meager in the vegetable department. Many contain around 300 calories, the amount of calories in one measly bagel. In order to make the entrées satisfying, I found myself adding vegetables, cooked rice or noodles, or grated cheese. And if people are eating them as their complete meal, they are also totally devoid of fruit. Most frozen entrées are going to be brimming with sodium. The companies taste-test products with the average American's taste preferences in mind, and the average American likes salt.

You can add an extra half cup of whole-grain noodles or brown rice, half cup of steamed vegetables, and a piece or two of fruit to help round out the entrées, which is what I did when I was trying each of the entrées listed on the following page. But this is sort of defeating the purpose of a frozen entrée, isn't it? I listed the nutrition information of some of the frozen entrees I found interesting in my supermarket. For some of the entrées that are begging for some added vegetables and starches, I provided two analysis—one with and one without the added foods.

Because some people with type 2 diabetes fare better with a little more fat in their meal (preferably monounsaturated fat), I included any non "light" entrée that seemed workable.

Brand/ Meal	Calories	Carbs (g)	Fat (g,%*)	Protein (g)	Fiber (g)	Sodium (mg)
Healthy Choice						
Chicken enchilada suiza	280	43	6 (19%)	14	5	440
Shrimp and vegetables	270	39	6 (20%)	15	6	80
Herb baked fish	340	54	7 (19%)	16	5	480
Traditional breast of turkey	290	40	4.5 (14%)	22	5	460
Chicken enchilada supreme	300	46	7 (21%)	13	4	560

Brand/ Meal	Calories	Carbs (g)	Fat (g,%*)	Protein (g)	Fiber (g)	Sodium (mg)
Lean Cuisine						
Chicken with basil	270	35	7 (23%)	16	3	580
Chicken in peanut sauce	290	35	6 (19%)	23	4	590
Baked fish with cheddar shells	270	36	5 (20%)	19	4	590
Fiesta chicken w/ black beans	290	40	4.5 (17%)	22	5	460
Cheese lasagna w/ chicken scallopini	290	33	8 (25%)	21	3	590
Shrimp and angel hair pasta	290	55	6 (19%)	10	1	590
3-bean chili	250	38	6 (22%)	10	9	590

Brand/ Meal	Calories	Carbs (g)	Fat (g,%*)	Protein (g)	Fiber (g)	Sodium (mg)
Budget Gourmet						
Three cheese lasagna	310	34	12 (35%)	15	2	700
Fettucini and meatballs in wine sauce with green beans	270	40	7 (23%)	15	3	560
Marie Calender's						
Chili and cornbread	540	67	21 (35%)	21	7	2,110
Sweet and sour chicken	570	86	15 (24%)	23	7	770
Beef tips in mushroom sauce	430	39	17 (36%)	25	6	1,620

Brand/ Meal	Calories	Carbs (g)	Fat (g,%*)	Protein (g)	Fiber (g)	Sodium (mg)
Marie Calender's						
Turkey with gravy	500	52	19 (34%)	31	4	2,040
Spaghetti and meat sauce	670	85	25 (34%)	31	9	1,160
Cheese ravioli in marinara sauce (w/ garlic bread)	750	96	29	25	1	1,070
Stuffed pasta trio	640	40	18 (25%)	15	5	950
Swanson						
Mexican style combo	470	59	18 (34%)	18	5	1,610
Chicken parmigiana	370	40	17 (41%)	13	4	1,010

Brand/ Meal	Calories	Carbs (g)	Fat (g,%*)	Protein (g)	Fiber (g)	Sodium (mg)
Swanson						
Herb roasted chicken breast tenders with rice and vegetables	310	4	7 (20%)	16	3	780
Turkey dinnner	310	40	8.5 (25%)	22	5	890

*Percent of calories from fat

Saturated fat for all items is between 1 and 9 mg.

Dairy products

We need milk to keep our cereal company, help liquefy our pancake batter, and lighten our coffee. The great thing about milk is you can take out some of the fat and saturated fat and still have milk that does all the things you want it to do. And as you remove the fat, the cholesterol goes too.

- Milk goes from 35 mg cholesterol in a cup of whole milk down to 15 mg in a cup of 1-percent milk.
- Cottage cheese goes from 25 mg cholesterol in a half cup of small curd cottage cheese down to 10 mg in low-fat.

- It gets a little tricky with other dairy products. When you take the fat out of cheese, for example, if you start going past the halfway mark, it starts looking and tasting a lot less like cheese and a lot more like plastic.

No matter what the amount of fat, most dairy products should be consumed in reasonable amounts; they all need to be counted into your daily totals, because many contribute carbohydrate grams galore, such as fat-free flavored yogurts. Then, the other dairy products that are low in carbohydrates need to be counted, because they are most likely contributing some fat grams (such as cheese). Either way, you want to make sure you are counting them in to see how they help balance your meals or snacks and what effect it has on your blood sugar in certain amounts.

Food	Calories	Carbs (g)	Fat (g)	Protein (g)	Fiber (g)	Sodium (mg)
Milk (1 cup)						
Skim milk	90	13	0	9	0	130
Low-fat milk (1%)	120	14	2.5	11	1.5	160
Low-fat milk (2%)	130	13	5	10	3	140
Whole milk	150	13	8	8	5	125

Food	Calories	Carbs (g)	Fat (g)	Protein (g)	Fiber (g)	Sodium (mg)
Cottage cheese (1/2 cup)						
Low-fat cottage cheese	80	3	2 (22%)	13	1	340
Small curd	120	4	5 (38%)	14	3	410
Yogurt						
"Light" fat-free, flavored 6-ounce yogurts	90	15	0	5	0	75
99% fat-free 6-ounce flavored	170	33	2	5	1	80
Low-fat custard style 6-ounce flavored	190	32	3	8	2	100

High-monounsaturated-fat salad dressings and spreads

The products listed here contain exclusively the high-monounsaturated-fat vegetable oils: canola oil, olive oil, or a combination of the two.

Food	Calories	Carbs (g)	Fat (g)
Mayonnaise: 1 Tablespoon*			
Safeway Select Real Mayonnaise with canola	0	0	11
Spectrum Canola Mayo	100	0	12
Spectrum Lite Canola Eggless Mayonnaise	35	1	3
Salad dressing: 2 Tablespoons**			
Kraft Special Collection			
Sun-Dried Tomato	60	4	4.5
Italian Pesto	70	5	5.5
Balsamic Vinaigrette	110	1	12
Kraft—Light Done Right			
Red Wine Vinaigrette	50	3	4.5
Italian	50	2	4.5
Raspberry Vinaigrette	60	6	4
Cucumber Ranch	60	2	5.5
Catalina	80	9	5
Kraft			
Roasted Garlic Vinaigrette	50	3	4.5

Food	Calories	Carbs (g)	Fat (g)
Kraft			
Ceasar Parmesian	60	1	5
Newman's Own			
Dynamite Lite Italian	45	3	4
Balsamic Vinaigrette	90	3	9
Berstein's			
Italian Cheese and Garlic	110	2	11
Red Wine and Garlic Italian	110	2	11
Parmesian Garlic Ranch	140	2	14
Balsamic Italian	110	2	11

*Mayonnaise: 80 or less mg sodium and 1 g saturated fat per serving.

**Salad dressing: Between 230 and 480 mg sodium and 1 g saturated fat per serving.

Chapter 7

Restaurant Rules to Eat By

Most health-conscious people go to restaurants and try to steer clear of one thing: overtly high-fat, high-calorie menu selections. But people with diabetes often have a few more things they worry about when approaching the menu. You need to get a feel for how many carbohydrate grams you might be eating and whether it is something that tends to keep your after-meal blood sugars high or not. You want to choose something that contributes a moderate amount of monounsaturated fat, because many find this helps with blood-sugar control. You will also be trying to keep saturated fat and trans fatty acids low and omega-3 fatty acids high, to help protect your heart. Many of you also need to count protein and potassium if you are on dialysis.

That's quite a bit to have on your plate (so to speak). All this could very well take the fun out of eating out, couldn't it? The trick is finding the happy medium between counting what you need to count and ordering and enjoying foods you like. It can be done. It takes a little practice. And having the grams of fat, fiber, and carbohydrate for various menu selections helps too. If your doctor or dietitian has told you to limit sodium, some of the suggested foods in this chapter have higher amounts of sodium than others, so make sure to consider that in choosing.

Cutting fat and calories when eating out

Remember that some people with diabetes control their blood sugar better if they aren't on a very low-fat diet, but are on a moderate-fat diet (around 30 to 35 percent of calories from fat). If you are in this group, it is particularly important that you choose monounsaturated fats and omega-3 and omega-9 fatty acids whenever possible. No matter which group you are in, though, you will want to avoid foods high in animal fats, which load on extra calories and saturated fat. One of the downfalls of eating out is the hefty portions of meat and dairy they often serve you. There are a few things you can do to keep this in check:

- The lean cuts of beef at restaurants are usually filet mignon, sirloin, sirloin tips, or chopped sirloin, while the fatter cuts are rib eye, prime rib, porterhouse, and T-bone.

- Make sure your "meat" dish is accompanied by lots of vegetables (beans when possible). The vegetables will help fill you up so you won't be tempted to overdo the meat, and the vegetables and beans help boost fiber totals too (good for your health and your blood sugars).

- Order the "kid size" burger or quarter-pounder instead of the third- or half-pound hamburger, and load up on lettuce, tomato, ketchup, and mustard, instead of mayonnaise, "special sauces," and cheese.

- Order the "petite" or "junior" portions of meat, prime rib, and steaks when available.

- Automatically cut your steak, pork chop, ham, or roasted chicken in half and take the rest home for tomorrow's sandwich.

- Ask the restaurant to make your "three-egg" omelet with egg substitute, or one egg blended with three egg whites.

- Avoid "extra cheese" and try to keep your servings of heavy cheese dishes (pizza, cheese enchiladas, lasagna, etc.) moderate.

To avoid excessive calories in general, you basically need to avoid ordering foods made with *lots* of:

- **Butter or margarine:** Each tablespoon of butter contains 11.5 grams fat and 102 calories.

- **Mayonnaise:** Each tablespoon of mayonnaise contains 11 grams of fat and 100 calories. Creamy mayonnaise-based salad dressings are dripping with fat grams. Remember one restaurant ladle adds up to two tablespoons of dressing, worth around 25 grams of fat.

- **Cream:** One-quarter cup of liquid whipping cream contains 22 grams fat and 205 calories.

- **Oil:** Each tablespoon of oil contains 14 grams fat and 120 calories. Avoid deep fried anything, even if it is something healthful such as chicken or seafood. Have it grilled instead.

- **Sugar:** It is loaded with calories. It's not that you can't have any. It helps to split the dessert you want to try with someone at the table or eat half and bring the other half home.

Restaurant chains menu picks

The steakhouse chain

There are many steakhouse chains across the country, and most of them do **not** provide any nutrition information for their interested patrons. Hopefully it's obvious to avoid the gigantic, battered, and deep-fried onion, which, rumor has it, contains more than 100 grams of fat.

Even if you avoid everything that is deep-fried (not just because of the fat and calories, but because anything deep-fried seems to cause high blood sugars for many people), what about the other items? If you want to have steak, which ones are best for you? There are few things, no matter which steakhouse you're in, that will help put you in the nutritional driver's seat:

• Ask that the chef cook your meat without butter or added fat.

• Order your meat in small portions or have the kitchen cut a large portion in half and put the second half immediately into a doggy bag.

• Order your baked potato with butter and sour cream on the side.

• Order your salad with the dressing on the side.

• Trim the visible chunks of fat from your steak before you eat it.

I did some investigating and came up with the nutrition information for some typical steakhouse menu items. The actual nutrition content of your particular steakhouse item might be higher in fat and calories, but the following information will get you in the ballpark.

Entrées

• **Grilled chicken:** 1 g carbohydrate, 2 g fat (15 percent of calories from fat), 25 g protein, 120 calories.

• **Grilled chicken sandwich:** 39 g carbohydrate, 4 g fat (11 percent of calories from fat), 33 g protein, 324 calories.

- **Grilled salmon (4 oz.):** 1 g carbohydrate, 10 g fat (42 percent of calories from fat), 34 g protein, 240 calories.

- **Sirloin tips with peppers and onions:** 4 g carbohydrate, 8 g fat (35 percent of calories from fat), 27 g protein, 203 calories.

- **Spicy BBQ chicken sandwich:** 45 g carbohydrate, 5 g fat (12 percent of calories from fat), 34 g protein, 368 calories.

- **Home-style chicken fillet:** 21 g carbohydrate, 9 g fat (37 percent of calories from fat), 13 g protein, 217 calories.

- **Junior sirloin steak:** 0 g carbohydrate, 10 g fat (46 percent of calories from fat), 25 g protein, 194 calories.

- **Filet mignon (5.5 oz. cooked):** 0 g carbohydrate, 15 g fat (44 percent of calories from fat), 44 g protein, 0 fiber, 330 calories.

- **Smothered steak sandwich:** 36 g carbohydrate, 15 g fat (31 percent of calories from fat), 34 g protein, 430 calories.

- **Sirloin steak:** 0 g carbohydrate, 16 g fat (51 percent of calories from fat), 34 g protein, 285 calories.

- **Country steak with gravy:** 44 g carbohydrate, 25 g fat (42 percent of calories from fat), 32 g protein, 530 calories.

Sides

- **Baked potato, plain:** 31 g carbohydrate, 0 g fat, 3 g protein, 3 g fiber, 130 calories.

- **Broccoli spears:** 5 g carbohydrate, 0 g fat, 33 g protein, 3 g fiber, 35 calories.

- **Corn (4 oz.)**: 28 g carbohydrate, 1.5 g fat (9 percent of calories from fat), 4 g protein, 3 g fat, 120 calories.

- **BBQ beans (4 oz.)**: 25 g carbohydrate, 2 g fat (14 percent of calories from fat), 6 g protein, 5 g fiber, 150 calories.

- **Rice pilaf (half cup)**: 23 g carbohydrate, 3.5 g fat (23 percent of calories from fat), 2 g protein, .5 g fiber, 135 calories.

- **Dinner roll (1)**: 14 g carbohydrate, 2 g fat (22 percent of calories from fat), 2g protein, 1 g fiber, 85 calories.

- **Cornbread (1 piece)**: 28 g carbohydrate, 5 g fat (26 percent of calories from fat), 4.5 g protein, 1.5 g fiber, 175 calories.

- **Cinnamon apples**: 34 g carbohydrate, 5 g fat (26 percent of calories from fat), 0 g protein, 2 g fiber, 172 calories.

- **Mashed potatoes (half cup)**: 18 g carbohydrate, 5 g fat (35 percent of calories from fat), 2 g protein, 2 g fiber, 115 calories.

- **Biscuit (1)**: 29 g carbohydrate, 15 g fat (50 percent of calories from fat), 5 g protein, 1 g fiber, 270 calories.

Soups (1 cup)

- **Vegetable beef**: 18 g carbohydrate, 2 g fat (15 percent of calories from fat), 7 g protein, 3 g fiber, 120 calories.

- **Clam chowder, New England**: 17 g carbohydrate, 9 g fat (45 percent of calories from fat), 3 g protein, 1.5 g fiber, 180 calories.

- **Chili with beans:** 25 g carbohydrates, 9 g fat (30 percent of calories from fat), 23 g protein, 5 g fiber, 270 calories.

Chili's

Chili's has a "Guiltless Grill" section in their menu, featuring four entrées ranging from 8 to 14 grams fat and 480 to 650 calories. All of these are really high in fiber too. The following selections have a good chance of fitting into your diabetic, carbo-counting eating plan.

- **Guiltless Grill Salmon:** 31 g carbohydrate, 14 g fat, 3 g saturated fat, 10 g fiber, 480 calories.

- **Guiltless Chicken Sandwich:** 63 g carbohydrate, 8 g fat, 2 g saturated fat, 11 g fiber, 490 calories.

- **Guiltless Chicken Platter:** 85 g carbohydrate, 9 g fat, 3 g saturated fat, 5 g fiber 580 calories. To reduce the grams of carbohydrate, eat less of the rice.

- **Guiltless Black Bean Burger:** 96 g carbohydrate, 12 g fat, 2 g saturated fat, 26 g fiber, 650 calories. To reduce the grams of carbohydrate from 96 to 48, eat half of the burger at the meal. If you need more food, add a nice green side salad with lots of vegetables and light dressing.

Good choices at pizza parlors

Some pizza chains have higher-fat pizza crust, while others have the more traditional, bread-type crust. I trust you can tell the difference. But in case you can't, lay your slice of pizza on a thick napkin. Do the grease spots form a triangle where the crust was? The grease from the crust is an indication of its fat content. It's best to frequent the pizza places that have the more traditional bread crusts—that's half the battle. Domino's, for example, makes a hand-tossed pizza crust and a pan crust. The hand-tossed is the one you want to ask for, because it has half the fat and saturated fat of deep-dish pizza.

The second factor in choosing the healthier pizza pie is the toppings—the cheese and all the trimmings. If you ask them to make the pizza with less cheese, this will definitely help. I know you feel silly doing this, but many of these restaurants really do put on more cheese than pizza really needs. If you are used to the typical sausage and pepperoni pizza, this next tip could be a tough one. If you top your pizza with items that don't add fat calories, but instead add nutrition and fiber, you are hitting the nutrition jackpot. You see, people usually don't have any vegetables with their pizza meal (unless they order a salad), so why not top your pizza with the vegetables you like and make it a more complete meal? Hopefully you like a couple of the following vegetable toppings: peppers, onions, mushrooms, zucchini, fresh tomatoes, broccoli, artichoke hearts, and also fruits such as pineapple. The leaner meat toppings are Canadian bacon and ham.

Blood sugar beware

Pizza seems to be one of those foods that raises blood sugar beyond what the grams of carbohydrate could explain. You might find you tolerate your pizza better if you have a side salad, heavy on the kidney beans, before you eat your pizza. This is probably not a good time to be eating a big slice of cake either. Try two large-size slices of cheese pizza and see how your blood sugar fares. Two slices will bring you to about 45 g of carbohydrate, 10 g of fat, 13 g of protein, 317 calories, and 669 mg sodium. Two deep-dish bring you to 54 g of carbohydrate, 20 g of fat, 18 g of protein, 455 calories, and 1,030 mg of sodium.

Good choices at sandwich shops

There are some really great choices at some sandwich restaurants. If you opt for the whole- or part-wheat selections, your grams of fiber might go up about 2 to 4 grams per sandwich. If you add mayonnaise or salad dressing, you'll need to add this into the equation. Good news though: Subway offers light mayonnaise. Other condiments available upon request are mustard, vinegar, and an olive oil blend.

Blimpie (per 6-inch sub)

- **Blimpie Best:** 47 g carbohydrate, 13 g fat (28 percent of calories from fat), 26 g protein, 4 g fiber, 410 calories, 1,480 mg sodium.

- **Ham and Swiss:** 47 g carbohydrate, 13 g fat (27 percent of calories from fat), 25 g protein, 5 g fiber, 430 calories, 970 mg sodium.

- **Turkey:** 51 g carbohydrate, 4.5 g fat (13 percent of calories from fat), 19 g protein, 3 g fiber, 320 calories, 690 mg sodium.

- **Roast Beef:** 47 g carbohydrate, 4.5 g fat (12 percent of calories from fat), 27 g protein, 2 g fiber, 340 calories, 870 mg sodium.

- **Club:** 53 g carbohydrate, 13 g fat (26 percent of calories from fat), 30 g protein, 3 g fiber, 450 calories, 1,350 mg sodium.

- **Grilled Chicken:** 52 g carbohydrate, 9 g fat (20 percent of calories from fat), 28 g protein, 2 g fiber, 400 calories, 960mg sodium.

- **Grilled Chicken Salad:** 13 g carbohydrate, 12 g fat (31 percent of calories from fat), 47 g protein, 0 g fiber, 350 calories, 1,190 mg sodium.

Subway Subs (per 6-inch sub)

- **Veggie Delite:** 44 g carbohydrates, 3 g fat (11 percent of calories from fat), 9 g protein, 237 calories, 593 mg sodium.

- **Turkey Breast:** 46 g carbohydrates, 4 g fat (12 percent of calories from fat), 18 g protein, 289 calories, 1,403 mg sodium.

- **Turkey Breast and Ham:** 46 g carbohydrate, 5 g fat (15 percent of calories from fat), 18 g protein, 295 calories, 1,361 mg sodium.

- **Ham:** 45 g carbohydrate, 5 g fat (15 percent of calories from fat), 19 g protein, 302 calories, 1,319 mg sodium.

- **Roast Beef:** 45 g carbohydrate, 5 g fat (15 percent of calories from fat), 20 g protein, 303 calories, 939 mg sodium.

- **Subway Club:** 46 g carbohydrate, 5 g fat (14 percent of calories from fat), 21 g protein, 312 calories, 1,352 mg sodium.

- **Seafood and Crab (made with light mayo):** 45 g carbohydrate, 10 g fat (26 percent of calories from fat), 20 g protein, 347 calories, 884 mg sodium.

- **Roasted Chicken Breast:** 47 g carbohydrate, 6 g fat (16 percent of calories from fat), 27 g protein, 348 calories, 978 mg sodium.

- **Steak and Cheese:** 47 g carbohydrate, 10 g fat (23 percent of calories from fat), 30 g protein, 398 calories, 1,117 mg sodium.

- **Subway Melt (includes cheese):** 46 g carbohydrate, 12 g fat (28 percent of calories from fat), 23 g protein, 382 calories, 1,746 mg sodium.

Subway Deli-Style Sandwiches (on deli-style roll)

- **Turkey:** 38 g carbohydrate, 4 g fat (15 percent of calories from fat), 12 g protein, 235 calories, 944 mg sodium.

- **Ham:** 37 g carbohydrate, 4 g fat (15 percent of calories from fat), 11 g protein, 234 calories, 773 mg sodium.

- **Roast Beef:** 38 g carbohydrate, 4 g fat (15 percent of calories from fat), 13 g protein, 245 calories, 638 mg sodium.

- **Tuna (with light mayo):** 38 g carbohydrate, 9 g fat (29 percent of calories from fat), 11 g protein, 279 calories, 583 mg sodium.

Subway Salads (not including dressing)

- **Veggie Delite:** 10 g carbohydrate, 1 g fat (18 percent of calories from fat), 2 g protein, 51 calories, 308 mg sodium.

- **Turkey Breast:** 12 g carbohydrate, 2 g fat (18 percent of calories from fat), 11 g of protein, 102 calories, 1,117 mg sodium.

- **Subway Club:** 12 g carbohydrate, 3 g fat (21 percent of calories from fat), 11 g protein, 126 calories, 1,067 mg sodium.

- **Roast Beef:** 11 g carbohydrate, 3 g fat (23 percent of calories from fat), 12 g protein, 117 calories, 654 mg sodium.

- **Ham:** 11 g carbohydrate, 3 g fat (23 percent of calories from fat), 12 g protein, 116 calories, 1,034 mg sodium.

- **Turkey Breast and Ham:** 11 g carbohydrate, 3 g fat (25 percent of calories from fat), 11 g protein, 109 calories, 1,076 mg sodium.

- **Roasted Chicken Breast:** 13 g carbohydrate, 4 g fat (22 percent of calories from fat), 20 g protein, 162 calories, 693 mg sodium.

- **Steak & Cheese:** 13 g carbohydrate, 8 g fat (34 percent of calories from fat), 22 g protein, 212 calories, 832 mg sodium

Good choices at fast-food chains

It's too easy to eat a horrendously high-fat, high-calorie meal at your average fast-food chain. Probably the biggest problems are that they are the heart-damaging types of fat, and you'd be hard pressed to find a fruit or vegetable to munch on. Some of the restaurants now offer side salads and fat-free or light salad dressing to go with your sandwich selection. If you know you will be eating fast food, bring along some fruit and raw vegetables (carrots or celery) to help round off the meal. I know this sounds totally impractical. But, if you eat fast food often, this is an important habit to get into.

When it comes to burgers, bigger is not better. The smaller the hamburger, the lower the percent of calories from fat. Some of this has to do with the smaller hamburgers having more bun per square inch of burger. But some of it has to do with the bigger burgers getting the fancier (and higher fat) sauces while the small burgers are served with catsup and mustard. Each fast-food chain has its pluses and minuses, but keep these three restaurant rules in mind:

1. Be cautious about your condiments

Half of the fat grams in Arby's Southwest Chicken Wrap and their Ultimate BLT Wrap come from the ranch sauce or mayonnaise.

Believe it! Some condiments add a lot of fat and calories such as mayonnaise-based sauces and oil-based sauces, while others are lower in calories and add no fat grams (but they will add some sodium). Choose to add a little catsup, marinara, mustard, or BBQ sauce instead of the creamy sauces and spreads. Half of a packet of BBQ sauce or honey mustard sauce from most fast-food chains, for example, will add about 23 calories, no fat grams, about 5 grams of carbohydrate, and about 80 milligrams of sodium.

2. Watch out for the side dishes

Anything on the side that's fried is suspect, such as french fries and onion rings. If you need something to keep your entrée company, look for fresh fruit cups or side salads (using half a packet of the reduced calorie dressings). The other option is to bring your own fruits and vegetables from home! Hey, don't laugh—I've done this plenty of times! These items will add some grams of carbohydrate to the meal, but they are also adding fiber and nutrients along with it.

3. Liquid calories add up

The last thing you need when eating a meal at a fast-food chain is to drink something that contributes calories and grams of carbohydrate without nutrients, such as soda, sweetened tea, lemonade, or fruit drinks. It's worse if it's loaded with fat grams in addition to sugar and calories, like shakes are! Choose a beverage that either contributes no calories (such as water, unsweetened tea, or diet soda) or a beverage that contributes some nutrients along with calories, such as low-fat milk or 100-percent orange juice. One carton of 1 percent low-fat milk will add 12 grams of carbohydrate to the meal. Eight ounces of 100-percent orange juice will add 22 grams of carbohydrate to the meal.

Keeping track of your carbohydrate, fiber, and fat grams

If you are keeping track of your carbohydrate, fiber, and fat grams to help you normalize your blood sugars, keep doing that, especially when you are eating at fast-food chains. All the nutrition information you will need can usually be found on the fast food-chain Website. BEFORE you go, look up the items you tend to want to order. Sometimes they will have a nutrition information pamphlet at the fast food restaurant or a poster with the information posted somewhere in the restaurant.

Now, with those three rules in mind, here are 21 alternatives to higher calorie, higher fat and saturated fat fare from fast-food chains.

Sandwiches

- **KFC Honey BBQ Sandwich:** 32 g carbohydrate, 3.5 g fat, 1 g saturated fat, 14 g protein, 3 g fiber, 280 calories, 780 mg sodium, 60 mg cholesterol.
- **KFC Tender Roast Sandwich without sauce:** 28 g carbohydrate, 4.5 g fat, 1.5 g saturated fat, 37 g protein, 2 g fiber, 300 calories, 1,060 mg sodium, 70 mg cholesterol.
- **Chick-fil-A Chargrilled Chicken Sandwich:** 33 g of carbohydrate, 3.5 g fat, 1 g saturated fat, 28 g protein, 3 g fiber, 270 calories, 940 mg sodium, 65 mg cholesterol.
- **Hardee's Charbroiled BBQ Chicken Sandwich:** 40 g carbohydrate, 4 g fat, 1 g saturated fat, 33 g of protein, 3 g fiber, 340 calories, 1,070 mg sodium, 60 mg cholesterol.

- Carl's Jr Charbroiled BBQ Chicken Sandwich: 48 g carbohydrate, 4.5 g fat, 1 g saturated fat, 34 g protein, 4 g fiber, 360 calories, 1150 mg sodium, 60 mg cholesterol.

- Wendy's Ultimate Grill Sandwich: 36 g carbohydrate, 7 g fat, 1.5 g saturated fat, 28 g protein, 2 g fiber, 320 calories, 950 mg sodium, 70 mg cholesterol.

- Arby's Grilled Chicken Cordon Bleu Sandwich (without mayo): 49 g carbohydrate, 8 g fat, 2 g saturated fat, 41 g protein, 2 g fiber, 390 calories, 1563 mg sodium, 25 mg cholesterol.

- In-n-Out Hamburger with onion, mustard, and ketchup instead of spread: 41 g carbohydrate, 10 g fat, 4 g saturated fat, 16 g protein, 3 g fiber, 310 calories, 730 mg sodium, 35 mg cholesterol.

Wraps and such

- Taco Bell Fresco Style Bean Burrito: 54 g carbohydrate, 7 g fat, 2.5 g saturated fat, 12 g protein, 9 g fiber, 330 calories, 1200 mg sodium, 0 mg cholesterol.

- KFC Oven Roasted Twister without sauce: 39 g carbohydrate, 7 g fat, 2.5 g saturated fat, 28 g protein, 3 g fiber, 330 calories, 1120 mg sodium, 50 mg cholesterol.

- McDonalds Grilled Snack Wrap with honey mustard (OR)

- Grilled Snack Wrap with chipotle BBQ sauce: 27 g carbohydrate, 8 g fat, 3.5 g saturated fat, 18 g protein, 1 g fiber, 260 calories, 820 mg sodium, 45 mg cholesterol.

- Taco Bell Fresco Style Steak Burrito Supreme: 48 g carbohydrate, 8 g fat, 3 g saturated fat, 16 g protein, 7 g fiber, 330 calories, 21,250 mg sodium, 0 mg cholesterol.

- Jack in the Box Chicken Fajita Pita (no salsa): 30 g carbohydrate, 9 g fat, 3.5 g saturated fat, 21 g protein, 2 g fiber, 280 calories, 1,110 mg sodium, 60 mg cholesterol.

- Chick-fil-A Chargrilled Chicken Cool Wrap: 46 g carbohydrate, 12 g fat, 3.5 g saturated fat, 34 g protein, 8 g fiber, 410 calories, 1,310 mg sodium, 70 mg cholesterol.

Entrée salads

- Chick-fil-A Chargrilled Chicken Garden Salad (without dressing): 9 g carbohydrate, 6 g fat, 3 g saturated fat, 22 g protein, 3 g fiber, 180 calories, 620 mg sodium, 65 mg cholesterol.

- Taco Bell Fresco Style Zesty Chicken Border Bowl (without dressing): 51 g carbohydrate, 8 g fat, 1.5 g saturated fat, 19 g protein, 10 g fiber, 350 calories, 1600 mg sodium, 25 mg cholesterol.

- McDonalds Southwest Salad with grilled chicken: 30 g carbohydrate, 9 g fat, 3 g saturated fat, 30 g protein, 7 g fiber, 320 calories, 970 mg sodium, 70 mg cholesterol.

- Arby's Martha's Vineyard Salad (without dressing): 24 g carbohydrate, 8 g fat, 4 g saturated fat, 26 g protein, 4 g fiber, 277 calories, 451 mg sodium, 72 mg cholesterol.

- Carl's Jr Charbroiled Chicken Salad (with low-fat balsamic dressing): 21 g carbohydrate, 8.5 g fat, 3.5 g saturated fat, 34 g protein, 5 g fiber, 295 calories, 1190 mg sodium, 75 mg cholesterol.

• **Arby's Santa Fe Salad with grilled chicken (without dressing):** 21 g carbohydrate, 9 g fat, 4 g saturated fat, 29 g protein, 6 g fiber, 283 calories, 521 mg sodium, 72 mg cholesterol.

• **McDonalds Asian Salad with grilled chicken:** 23 g carbohydrate, 10 g fat, 1 g saturated fat; 32 g protein, 5 g fiber, 300 calories, 890 mg sodium, 65 mg cholesterol.

Best and worst fast-food breakfasts

Results from a recent University of Minnesota study that noted breakfast habits and weight changes in 2,200 teens over a five-year period, indicated that regular breakfast eaters tended to have the lowest body mass indexes (BMIs) in a dose-response manner. In other words, as breakfast skipping frequency went up, so did the body mass indexes of these teens.

Eating breakfast is definitely "good," but if you do end up eating your breakfast at a fast-food chain, remember there are more healthful foods to be had.

In general, "studies show that some people tend to consume more calories, fat, and sodium, and fewer vitamins, on the days when they go to fast-food restaurants than on the days they don't," says Karen Collins, MS, RD, CDN, of the American Institute for Cancer Research.

One reason for this, she says, may be because our bodies don't automatically sense that we need smaller portions when we eat foods high in calories. "Not everyone is able to compensate by eating less later in the day," explains Collins.

In search of a better breakfast

Of course, some fast-food offerings are better than others. Finding a healthier breakfast means looking for items with some fiber and protein (which makes them more satisfying), but not too much saturated fat or total fat. Fiber is important for baked offerings too; even when these items are relatively low in fat, they can be high in sugar and white flour.

A look at the nutrition information some popular fast-food chains provide on their Web sites shows that few of their breakfast items fit the bill. Some offer one or two items that are reasonably low in fat and saturated fat and contain some protein, but they're usually lacking in fiber. Others have not even one main-dish breakfast item that's low enough in fat and saturated fat to be considered healthy. At Carl's Jr., for example, there was only one main-dish item with less than 20 grams of fat per serving (the French Toast Dips with 18 grams of fat and 2.5 grams saturated fat). It does contribute 9 grams of protein, but is lacking in the fiber department, with only 1 gram. Their worst choice on the breakfast menu is the Carl's Jr. Loaded Breakfast Burrito with 820 calories, 51 grams of fat, 16 grams of saturated fat, 595 milligrams of cholesterol, and 1,530 milligrams of sodium.

No matter which fast-food chain you visit, though, high-fat and high-calorie breakfast choices abound. When you find yourself at a fast-food or quick-serve chain before 11 a.m., choose a better breakfast option, keep your portions reasonable, and keep (or start!) exercising.

Starbucks Coffee (Bakery items vary regionally)

- **Low-Fat Bran Muffin:** 74 g carbohydrate, 4.5 g fat, 9 g protein, 7 g fiber, 360 calories, 290 mg sodium, 40 mg cholesterol.

- **Reduced-Fat Cranberry Apple Muffin:** 54 g carbohydrate, 9 g fat, 7 g protein, 5 g fiber, 310 calories, 460 mg sodium, 260 mg cholesterol.

- **Vegan Fruit Scone with Pecans:** 60 g carbohydrate, 5 g fat, 7 g protein, 3 g fiber, 310 calories, 320 mg sodium, 0 g cholesterol.

- **Spinach, Roasted Tomato, Feta, and Egg Wrap:** 29 g carbohydrate, 10 g fat, 13 g protein, 7 g fiber, 240 calories, 730 mg sodium, 140 mg cholesterol.

- **Reduced-Fat Blueberry Coffee Cake:** 54 g carbohydrate, 6 g fat, 4 g protein, 1 g fiber, 320 calories, 390 mg sodium, 10 mg cholesterol.

- **Reduced-Fat Cinnamon Swirl Coffee Cake:** 53 g carbohydrate, 6 g fat, 4 g protein, 1 g fiber, 300 calories, 370 mg sodium, 10 mg cholesterol.

McDonald's

- **Egg McMuffin:** 30 g carbohydrate, 12 g fat, 18 g protein, 2 g fiber, 300 calories, 820 mg sodium, 260 mg cholesterol.

- **Hotcakes (without syrup and margarine):** 60 g carbohydrate, 9 g fat, 8 g protein, 3 g fiber, 350 calories, 590 mg sodium, 20 mg cholesterol.

Burger King

- **Ham Omelet Sandwich:** 33 g carbohydrate, 13 g fat, 13 g protein, 1 g fiber, 290 calories, 870 mg sodium, 85 mg cholesterol.

- **French Toast Sticks (3 pieces):** 26 g carbohydrate, 13 g fat, 4 g protein, 1 g fiber, 240 calories, 260 mg sodium, 0 mg cholesterol.

Jack in the Box

- **Breakfast Jack:** 29 g carbohydrate, 12 g fat, 17 g protein, 1 g fiber, 290 calories, 760 mg sodium, 220 mg cholesterol.

- **Bacon Breakfast Jack:** 29 g carbohydrate, 14 g fat, 16 g protein, 1 g fiber, 300 calories, 730 mg sodium, 215 mg cholesterol.

Subway

- **Cheese Breakfast Sandwich (on 6-inch bread):** 55 g carbohydrate, 18 g fat, 30 g protein, 5 g fiber, 420 calories, 1,010 mg sodium, 190 mg cholesterol.

Bagel shops

I love fresh bagels! Spread with light cream cheese, they are one of my favorite breakfasts. Bagels look innocent enough, but they can be trouble for some people with diabetes. There's something about those 40-ish grams of carbohydrates that seems to make normal blood sugars difficult first thing in the morning for many people with type 2 diabetes. But there are a few things you can do to try to improve your post-bagel blood sugars.

Try whole-grain bagels or oat-bran bagels to see if that makes a difference. And make sure you balance your mostly carbohydrate bagel with some protein and a little fat. You can do this by spreading your bagel with light cream cheese or filling a savory bagel with some reduced-fat cheese and a slice of turkey breast. Here is how some of these options add up.

- **Whole grain/wheat bagel with 1 ounce reduced-fat cheese and 1 ounce roasted turkey breast:** 55 g carbohydrate, 8 g fat, 23 g protein, 9 g fiber, 375 calories, 842 mg sodium, 30 mg cholesterol.

- Whole grain/wheat bagel with 2 tablespoons light cream cheese: 54 g carbohydrate, 5.5 g fat, 14 g protein, 9 g fiber, 313 calories, 583 mg sodium, 13 mg cholesterol.

Chapter 8

Smart Snacking and Balanced Breakfasts

There are two specific areas of eating that Certified Diabetes Educators wanted me to give some extra information about: smart snacking and eating balanced breakfasts. So with all the information in this book behind you, here are two last ways you can help bring on better blood sugars.

Smart snacking

Do the words *chips, cookies, ice cream, candy bars,* or *crackers* mean anything to you? These higher-calorie, fat, or sugar foods represent our more popular snack foods. But to start snacking wisely, you don't necessarily need to trade all your Chips Ahoy cookies for carrot sticks, or your carton of ice cream for a carton of tofu. We can make smarter snack choices by choosing foods that are higher in fiber and important nutrients, feature carbohydrates with lower glycemic indexes, and that are balanced with some protein and some of the more heart-helpful fats.

Some people with diabetes need to eat snacks to help prevent low blood-glucose levels (mostly people with type 1 diabetes).

These healthful snacks can be eaten before going to bed, exercising, or at other times when hypoglycemia tends to strike. For the people with diabetes who are more at risk of having high blood sugars (hyperglycemia), which is most people with type 2 diabetes, smart snacks would include higher-fiber, lower-glycemic index ingredients.

Soluble fiber snacks

Foods rich in soluble fiber make for great snacks because soluble fiber leaves the stomach slowly, encouraging better blood sugars and making you feel satisfied longer. Here are some possible snack ingredients that are high in soluble fiber:

- **Peas and beans:** These include canned vegetarian or fat-free refried beans, green salad with canned kidney beans added, three-bean salad made with a light vinaigrette salad dressing.

- **Oats and oat bran:** Examples are low-sugar hot oatmeal, low-sugar oat or oat bran muffin, or low-sugar oat breakfast cereal.

- **Barley:** It can be found in a barley and vegetable soup or stew,

- **Some fruits:** Fruits such as apples, peaches, citrus, mango, plums, kiwi, pears, and berries can be blended in a smoothie, enjoyed with a whole grain low-sugar cereal, or mixed in plain or light yogurt.

- **Some vegetables:** These include artichokes, celery root, sweet potatoes, parsnips, turnips, acorn squash, brussels sprouts, cabbage, green peas, broccoli, carrots, cauliflower, asparagus, and beets.

Adding other plant foods that contribute some fat and/or protein into our snack recipes, such as nuts, soy foods, olive and canola oil, and avocado, may also help minimize high blood sugars resulting from traditionally high-carbohydrate snacks.

To help you practice smarter snacking and encourage better blood sugars, here are six more tips and recipes!

1. Whole grain snacks are a step in the right direction.

The latest research suggests that people who eat whole grains have the lowest incidence of diabetes. They appear to increase the efficiency of insulin so that less is required to metabolize the sugar.

After speaking with a few bagel-lovers, I thought I would calculate how to make a better bagel snack. Bagels are mostly carbohydrates, so it is important to top them with something that will add some protein and fat into the snack equation. This will make the bagel more satisfying, and the energy will hit the bloodstream more slowly and last longer. This topping could be a little bit of peanut butter, some light cream cheese, or a slice of reduced-fat cheese and a slice of turkey breast.

The other key to a better bagel snack is eating whole wheat or whole grain. This will pump some fiber into the picture and whole grains also contribute vitamin and minerals and phytochemicals that you aren't getting in bagels made with refined flour.

 ## Bagel and Cream Cheese

Makes 1 bagel snack.

- 1/2 whole wheat or whole grain bagel, toasted or untoasted
- 1 Tbs. of light cream cheese

Per serving: 108 calories, 2.7 g fiber, 4.5 g protein, 16.5 g carbohydrate, 2.9 g fat, 1.8 g saturated fat, 7.5 mg cholesterol, 210 mg sodium. Calories from fat: 24 percent.

2. Some foods do not cause high blood sugar.

Even in large amounts and if eaten alone, the following foods are not likely to result in a substantial rise in blood sugar:

- Meat.
- Poultry.
- Fish.
- Avocados.
- Salad vegetables.
- Cheese.
- Eggs.

(Foster-Powell et al., "International table of lycemic index and glycemic load values." *Am J Clin Nutr* 76 [2002]: 5–56)

 ## Mini Turkey Melts

This is a snack I make for my daughter and myself often. It works well with the toaster oven.

Makes 2 snack servings.

- 10 Triscuits
- 5 thin slices of turkey breast cut in half
- 2 oz. shredded, reduced-fat cheese of choice (Jarlsberg Lite, cheddar, jack)

1. Place 10 Triscuits in a toaster oven pan. Top each with half a slice of turkey (fold it over to fit).
2. Top the turkey with shredded cheese.
3. Broil in toaster oven, watching carefully, until cheese is nicely melted.

Per serving: 214 calories, 21 g protein, 16 g carbohydrate, 7 g fat (3.5 g saturated fat, 2.2 g monounsaturated fat, .1 g polyunsaturated fat), 40 mg cholesterol, 2 g fiber, 260 mg sodium (not including the sodium from the turkey; the sodium in turkey slices vary greatly by brand). Calories from fat: 29 percent.

3. Low glycemic index foods are less refined.

Low glycemic index foods are generally less refined than their higher glycemic index counterparts. For example, white bread has a glycemic index of 105 and a glycemic load of 10, while Healthy Choice Hearty 7 Grain bread has a glycemic index of 79 and a glycemic load of 8. Corn flakes has a glycemic index of 130 and a glycemic load of 24, while Raisin Bran cereal has a glycemic index of 87 (plus or minus 7) and a glycemic load of 12.

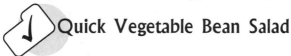

Quick Vegetable Bean Salad

One serving of this quick salad gives you a dose of alpha and beta carotene, folic acid, vitamin C, fiber, and plant omega-3 fatty acids from the canola oil. If you want to make this more of a meal, stir in a can of albacore tuna to add fish omega-3 fatty acids and some protein into the picture.

Makes 8 servings.

- 3 cups baby carrots, diced or thinly sliced
- 3 cups broccoli florets cut into bite-sized pieces
- 1 15-oz. can kidney beans, rinsed and drained well
- 1/2 cup finely chopped mild onion (use less if desired)
- 1/2 cup "1/3 less fat" bottled vinaigrette made with canola or olive oil. (I use Seven Seas 1/3 less fat Red Wine Vinaigrette with canola)
- 1 6-oz. can albacore tuna in water (optional)

1. Combine carrot pieces with 1/4 cup water in a microwave-safe covered dish and cook on high about three to five minutes (or until just barely tender). Drain well and add to medium-sized serving bowl.

2. Combine broccoli pieces with 1/4 cup water in a microwave-safe covered dish and cook on high about three to five minutes (or until just barely tender). Drain well and add to medium-sized serving bowl.

3. Add beans, chopped onion, and vinaigrette (and tuna if desired) to serving bowl. Toss well to blend.

Per serving: 110 calories, 5 g protein, 19 g carbohydrate, 2.5 g fat, 0 g saturated fat, 0 mg cholesterol, 7 g fiber, 310 mg sodium. Calories from fat: 20 percent.

4. Go ahead, get nutty.

An ounce of most nuts will add about 170 calories (with around 7 grams carbohydrate, 6 grams protein, and 15 grams fat). Which nuts are best? Hazelnuts and almonds are lowest in saturated fat, with macadamia and hazelnuts being the highest in monounsaturated fat (this is a good thing). Pistachios and macadamia nuts were highest in fiber (about 3 grams per ounce) with walnuts scoring highest in omega-3 fatty acids.

 Peanut Butter Banana Fana

Makes 2 snack servings.

- 1 banana
- 2 Tbs. smooth peanut butter (reduced-fat can also be used)
- Topping to roll banana in, such as cake-decorating sprinkles or Rice Krispies cereal.

1. Peel banana. Place on piece of foil and freeze for 1 hour. Remove peanut butter from refrigerator and bring to room temperature (so it's more spreadable).
2. Using a dinner knife, spread the peanut butter all around the banana.
3. Roll in food topping of choice, such as 1/2 cup of Rice Krispies cereal.
4. Place on foil sheet and refrigerate for 1 hour. It's ready to eat!

Per serving (with Rice Krispies cereal): 175 calories, 5.5 g protein, 22 g carbohydrate, 8 g fat, 1 g saturated fat, 0 mg cholesterol, 2.4 g fiber, 55 mg sodium. Calories from fat: 42 percent.

5. Yodel for yogurt.

A container of light fruit yogurt (low-fat and with artificial sweeteners) is a great snack at work or on the go. A 7-ounce container has about 13 grams of available carbohydrates and a glycemic index of 20, adding up to a glycemic load of only 2! Even the regular fruit yogurts (with added sugar) have about 31 grams of available carbohydrate (per 7 ounces) and a glycemic index of 47, adding up to a glycemic load of 10.

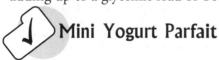# Mini Yogurt Parfait

Yogurt makes a great snack, but day after day it can get a bit boring. One way to make it a little more interesting is to make a parfait with layers of yogurt, fresh fruit, and low-fat granola. Here's one way to do this.

Makes 1 parfait.

Layer half of each of the following ingredients in a parfait glass, then repeat with the other half.

- 1/4 cup fresh fruit (such as berries or sliced peaches)
- 1/4 cup low-fat or regular yogurt (flavor of your choice)
- 1/4 cup low-fat granola

Per parfait: 160 calories, 5 g protein, 32 g carbohydrate, 2.5 g fat, 0.4 g saturated fat, 3 mg cholesterol, 2.6 g fiber, 80 mg sodium, 96 mg calcium. Calories from fat: 12 percent.

6. Enjoy portable fruit.

Fruit can travel well in your car or briefcase and comes in handy for a quick pick-me-up. Many fruits offer just enough carbohydrates with a nice dose of fiber. The following fruits have a low glycemic load (5 or less per serving):

- Cherries, glycemic load of 3 per (4 1/4 ounce) serving.
- Grapefruit, glycemic load of 3 per (4 1/4 ounce) serving.
- Kiwi fruit, glycemic load of 5 per (4 1/4 ounce) serving.
- Oranges, glycemic load of 5 per (4 1/4 ounce) serving.
- Peaches (fresh or canned in juice), glycemic load of 4 per (4 1/4 ounce) serving.
- Pears, glycemic load of 4 per (4 1/4 ounce) serving.
- Plums, glycemic load of 3 per (4 1/4 ounce) serving.
- Cantaloupe, glycemic load of 4 per (4 1/4 ounce) serving.
- Strawberries, glycemic load of 1 per (4 1/4 ounce) serving.

Melon Medley

Chilled melon is a refreshing afternoon or evening snack. Make a bowl of melon cubes or balls, cover the bowl, and keep it in the refrigerator for a quick snack.

Makes 4 snack servings.

- 3 cups honeydew melon balls or cubes
- 3 cups cantaloupe balls or cubes

In serving bowl, toss melon to mix.

Per serving: 87 calories, 1.6 g protein, 21.8 g carbohydrates, 0.5 g fat, 0 g saturated fat, 0 mg cholesterol, 1.7 g fiber, 23 mg sodium. Calories from fat: 4 percent.

Other snack suggestions

Pear and Jarlsberg Lite

This is one of my favorite snacks, pairing pear wedges with a nicely flavored cheese such as Jarlsberg Lite or Gruyere. What a great way to work another fruit serving into my day!

Per serving (1 sliced pear with 1 ounce of sliced Jarlsberg Lite): 202 calories, 9 grams protein, 32.5 g carbohydrate, 5.5 g fat (3 g saturated fat, 1.6 g monounsaturated fat, 0.3 g polyunsaturated fat), 15 mg cholesterol, 5 g fiber, 150 mg sodium, Calories from fat: 24 percent.

Healthy Pop Jolly Time popcorn

You knew it was coming. Sooner or later I would have to list microwave popcorn as a snack! The microwave popcorn companies usually use partially hydrogenated oils in their products, so you can bet many of the fat grams listed per serving are trans fatty acids. The less fat in the popcorn, the lower the amount of trans fatty acids!

All you need is a popcorn packet and a microwave—at home, at work, or even at the swim club—and you are good to go.

There are a few brands with a 94-percent fat free (or thereabouts) microwave popping corn. I'm going to give you the nutritional analysis for Jolly Time's Healthy Pop Butter Flavor Microwave Pop Corn—mainly because it's the type my daughters seem to like.

Per serving (5 cups popped—about 2 1/2 servings per bag): 90 calories, 2 grams fat, 2 grams saturated fat, 0 mg cholesterol, 210 mg sodium, 23 grams carb, 9 grams dietary fiber, and 4 grams protein.

Wendy's Side Salad

I found myself in the Wendy's drive-through recently ordering side salads for me and my girls, as we were rushing to the orthodontist and all in need of an afternoon snack. It's actually a fresh and colorful salad, and, best of all, it's on the 99-cent menu!

Per serving: (side salad dressed with half of a packet—2.5 ounces total—of reduced-fat creamy ranch dressing): 90 calories, 10.5 g carbohydrate, 2.5 g protein, 4.5 g fat, 0.7 g saturated fat, 7 mg cholesterol, about 2.5 g fiber, and 325 mg sodium.

Balanced breakfasts

If you normally eat dinner at 7 p.m., breakfast the next day is the first food your body has had in about 11 hours. When we put it that way, breakfast sure sounds important to the body's functioning doesn't it?

It's better health-wise to eat breakfast than to not eat breakfast…but it's definitely best to eat a balanced, nutrient-rich, higher fiber breakfast than one that is full of refined grains, sugar, salt, and/or saturated fat whether or not you have type 2 diabetes!

To eat breakfast or not eat breakfast? That is the question.

Some people may think skipping breakfast is a good way to trim calories and lose weight, but recent studies suggest the exact opposite. New research suggest the daily act of eating breakfast may decrease our risk of obesity, even after researchers controlled for other dietary factors and physical activity.

To maintain good health and prevent those hard-to-lose pounds from creeping on in the first place, make it a habit to eat a balanced breakfast. Many people go wrong by eating a breakfast with mostly refined carbohydrates and very little fiber and protein—such as a refined flour bagel or a muffin made with sugar and white flour, or a sugary low-fiber breakfast cereal. For a more satisfying meal, balancing carbohydrates (preferably from whole grains, fruit, and vegetables) with some protein and a little smart fat will do a better job of staving off hunger until lunch and fueling your entire morning's activities.

One quick tip I use to keep my breakfast balanced is to "strive for 5!" I try to include at least 5 grams of fiber and 5 grams of protein in every breakfast.

Strive for at least 5 grams of protein

Lower fat or nonfat dairy products will add protein to your breakfast, along with egg white or egg substitute (egg yolk doesn't contribute protein), lean breakfast meat options (Canadian bacon or extra lean ham, turkey bacon, light turkey sausage), and soy milk and soy products.

Breakfast Protein Options

Protein Options	Protein	Calories	Fat	Sat. Fat	Carbs
Skim milk, 1 cup	10	100	0	0	4
low-fat yogurt, vanilla, 1 cup	9.3	253	4.6	2.6	6
low-fat cottage cheese, 1 cup	28	160	2	1	6
reduced-fat cheese, 1 ounce	8	70	4	2.5	1
egg whites, 2	7	33	0	0	1
egg substitute (1.5 oz.)	6	30	0	0	1
soymilk, low-fat, 1 cup	4	90	1.5	0	14
soy-based sausage, 2 ounces	12	119	4.5	0.7	6
tofu, extra firm, light, 2 ounces	5	43	1.4	0	2.2
Canadian bacon, 2 ounces	12	89	3.9	1.2	1
extra-lean ham, 2 ounces	11	61	1.5	0.4	0.4
turkey bacon, 2 strips	4	70	6	2	0.1
light turkey sausage, 2 ounces	9	130	10	2.2	1
peanut butter, natural, 1 Tbs.	3.5	100	8	1	3.5

Breakfast Protein Options

Protein Options	Protein	Calories	Fat	Sat. Fat	Carbs
light cream cheese, 1 ounce	3	53	4	2.7	1.8
lox (smoked salmon), 1 ounce	5.2	33	1.2	0.2	0

Strive for at least 5 grams of fiber

One way to get to those five grams of fiber is to include a whole grain and/or fruit or vegetables with breakfast. I look for opportunities to switch to whole grains, because of the plethora of health benefits they offer, and breakfast is the perfect time to work in a serving or two. Whole grains offer a myriad of vitamins, minerals, and phytochemicals that together are likely to have significant health benefits beyond the fiber. New research suggests that eating whole grains may help reduce your risk of cardiovascular disease and certain cancers and for developing type 2 diabetes by improving insulin sensitivity, improving serum lipid levels, and by lowering oxidative stress.

Get your grains at breakfast by choosing from the following:

- Hot oatmeal (or another hot whole grain cereal).
- Cold whole-grain cereal.
- 100-percent whole wheat bread/toast, small bagel or English muffin, or tortilla.
- Pancakes and waffles made with at least half whole wheat flour plus oats, oat bran, or ground flaxseed added sometimes as well.
- Muffins and cinnamon rolls made with at least half whole wheat flour plus oats, oat bran, or ground flaxseed.

Weekend breakfast tip

If you have extra whole grain waffles, pancakes, muffins, etc. from the weekend, just freeze them in individual plastic bags for part of a quick breakfast during the week. Just pop them from the freezer into the microwave or toaster/toaster oven.

Other foods that help add fiber come from the plant food groups: fruits, vegetables, other whole grains, beans, and nuts.

Breakfast Fiber Options

Fiber Options	Fiber	Calories	Carbs	Fat	Protein
Grains					
oatmeal, cooked, 3/4 cup	3	124	21	2.7	4.5
whole-grain cereal, 1 cup	7	190	45	1.5	4
whole-wheat bread, 1 slice	2	70	14	1	3
whole-wheat bagel	9	260	52	1.5	11
whole-wheat torilla	8	300	54	4.5	12
whole-wheat flour, 1/4 cup	4	110	23	0	14
oats, rolled quick, 1/4 cup	2.3	83	14	1.5	3
barley med. cooked, 1/2 cup	5	220	55	0.7	5

Breakfast Fiber Options

Fiber Options	Fiber	Calories	Carbs	Fat	Protein
barley, pearl, cooked 1/2 cup	3	97	22	0.3	2
buckwheat groats, cooked, 1/2 cup	2.3	77	17	0.5	2.8
quinoa, cooked, 1/2 cup	2.6	111	20	1.8	4
Fruit					
banana, 1	3.1	105	27	0.4	1.3
bluberries, fresh, 1/2 cup	2	42	11	0.2	0.6
raspberries, fresh, 1/2 cup	4	32	7	0.4	0.7
dried fruit, mixed, 1/4 cup	2	120	28	0	1
melon, 2 cups (cantaloupe or honeydew)	3	108	26	0.3	3
Vegetables					
mushrooms, cooked, 1/2 cup	2	22	4	0.4	2
onions, cooked, 1/2 cup	2	29	7	0.1	1
zucchini, cooked, 1 cup	2.2	26	5	0.2	2
tomatoes, 1 med.	1	25	5	0	1

Breakfast Fiber Options

Fiber Options	Fiber	Calories	Carbs	Fat	Protein
Ground flaxseed, 2 Tbs.	3	80	4	6	3
pecans (or chopped nuts), 1/4 cup	3	205	4	21	3

Seven balanced breakfast examples with 50 grams of carbohydrate or less!

1. Omelet made with 1/2 cup egg substitute, 1/2 cup vegetables, 1 ounce reduced-fat cheese served on 100-percent whole grain English muffin. (288 calories, **35 g carbohydrate**, 7 g fiber, 28 g protein, 6 g fat, 2.5 g saturated fat, 15 mg cholesterol, 724 mg sodium.)

2. Multigrain waffle topped with 1/2 cup fresh fruit and 1/4-cup plain yogurt, with 1/8 teaspoon vanilla extract and a pinch of ground cinnamon stirred in. (265 calories, **48 g carbohydrate**, 8 g fiber, 11 g protein, 5 g fat, 1 g saturated fat, 12 mg cholesterol, 386 mg sodium.)

3. Two slices French toast made with whole grain bread and one higher omega-3 egg blended with 1/4 cup fat free half-and-half or low-fat milk plus 1/8 teaspoon vanilla and a pinch of ground cinnamon. (278 calories, **42 g carbohydrate**, 5 g fiber, 14 g protein, 6.5 g fat, 1.5 g saturated fat, 215 mg cholesterol, 480 mg sodium.)

4. Breakfast burrito made with 1 whole wheat tortilla (about 50 grams in weight per tortilla), 1/2 cup egg substitute scrambled with 1/2 cup assorted cooked vegetables, and 1-ounce of reduced-fat cheese. (304 calories, **32 g carbohydrate**, 6 g fiber, 25 g protein, 7 g fat, 2.5 g saturated fat, 15 mg cholesterol, 669 mg sodium.)

5. Homemade breakfast muffin sandwich made with 1 whole grain English muffin, 1 1/2-ounces light turkey breakfast sausage and 1 ounce reduced-fat cheese. (300 calories, **28 g carbohydrate**, 5 g fiber, 21 g protein, 12 g fat, 4 g saturated fat, 83 mg cholesterol, 690 mg sodium.)

6. Smoothie made with 6 ounces low-fat yogurt blended with 1 cup frozen fruit and 1/2 cup soymilk or low-fat milk. (230 calories, **42 g carbohydrate**, 6.5 g fiber, 9 g protein, 4 g fat, 1 g saturated fat, 5 mg cholesterol, 130 mg sodium.)

7. Yogurt breakfast parfait made with 6 ounces flavored low-fat yogurt, 1/2 cup fresh fruit (such as raspberries), topped with 1/8 cup nuts (such as walnuts), and 1/2-cup whole grain cereal (such as Grape Nut flakes). (300 calories, **44 g carbohydrate**, 7 g fiber, 10 g protein, 9.3 g fat, 0 g saturated fat, 0 mg cholesterol, 179 mg sodium]

Sources:

Nutritional Analysis by ESHA Research Food Processor SQL.

Smith Edge M. et al. "A New Life for Whole Grains." *Journal of the American Dietetic Association* 105, no. 12 (December 2005): 1856–1860.

Timlin M.T. et al. "Breakfast Eating and Weight Change in a 5-Year Prospective Analysis of Adolescents: Project EAT" *Pediatrics* 121, no. 3 (March 2008): e638–e645.

Bonus breakfast recipes

Strawberry Summer Muffins

These muffins are delicious fresh from the oven. If you are in the habit of spreading butter or margarine on your muffins, try some light cream cheese instead.

Makes 11 muffins (5.5 servings when 2 muffins each)

- 1 1/3 cup sliced fresh strawberries (frozen can also be used)
- 1/4 cup low-fat milk
- 1 teaspoon vanilla extract
- 1/2 teaspoon strawberry or raspberry extract (optional)
- 1/2 teaspoon red food coloring (optional)
- 1/4 cup reduced-fat margarine with the least amount of saturated/trans fat (with about 8 grams of fat per tablespoon)
- 1/2 cup granulated sugar (add 1/4 cup more sugar or Splenda if you prefer it sweeter)
- 1 large egg, room temperature (higher omega-3 if available)
- 1/4 cup egg substitute or 2 egg whites
- 1 cup whole wheat flour
- 1/2 cup unbleached white flour
- 1 teaspoon baking powder
- 1/4 teaspoon salt
- 1 tablespoon powdered sugar for dusting the tops (optional)

1. Preheat oven to 350 degrees. Line a 12-cup muffin tin with cupcake liners; set aside. Place strawberries in a small food processor; process until pureed. Make sure you have 2/3 cup of puree.

2. In a small bowl, combine 2/3 cup strawberry puree with low-fat milk, vanilla extract, strawberry extract and red food coloring (if desired); set aside.

3. In the bowl of an electric mixer fitted with the paddle attachment, cream margarine and sugar on medium-high speed until combined and fluffy. Reduce speed to medium-low and add the egg and egg substitute or egg white, beating just until blended. Make sure to scrape the side and bottom of bowl well halfway through.

4. With mixer turned off, in medium bowl, whisk together flours, baking powder, and salt then add half of the flour mixture to the mixing bowl with margarine mixture, beating just until blended. Pour in the strawberry mixture and beat on low just until blended, scraping sides of bowl with spatula midway. Add in the remaining flour mixture, beating just until blended and scraping down sides of the bowl.

5. Add 1/4 cup of muffin batter to each prepared muffin cup. Bake until tops are just dry to the touch (about 22 minutes). Let cool completely in tin before dusting with powdered sugar if desired.

Per 2 muffin serving: 258 calories, 8 g protein, 47 g carbohydrate, 6 g fat, 1 g saturated fat, 40 mg cholesterol, 4 g fiber, 260 mg sodium. Calories from fat: 20 percent.

Veggie Microwave Frittata

This is a tasty breakfast dish for two made in about 10 minutes. You can garnish each serving with fresh chopped tomato or salsa and/or avocado wedges.

Makes 2 servings

- 1 1/4 cup shredded fat-free frozen hash browns
- 2/3 cup shredded or grated carrot
- 1/4 cup chopped onion
- 1 tablespoon chopped fresh parsley (or 1 1/2 teaspoon parsley flakes)
- 2 teaspoons olive oil or canola oil
- pinch salt and pepper (optional)
- 2 large eggs (higher omega-3 fatty acids if available)
- 1/2 cup egg substitute
- 1/4 cup low-fat milk or fat-free half-and-half
- 1/8 teaspoon dry mustard
- two dashes hot pepper sauce (such as Tabasco)
- 1/2 cup shredded reduced-fat sharp cheddar cheese

1. In a microwave-safe 1-quart casserole dish, combine potatoes, carrot, onion, parsley, and oil. Cover and microwave on high for three minutes, stirring after 90 seconds. Add salt and pepper if desired.

2. In mixing bowl, combine eggs, egg substitute, milk, mustard, and hot pepper sauce by beating on medium speed for a minute or two. Pour egg mixture into casserole dish and stir to combine with potato mixture.

3. Cover dish (waxed paper will work) and microwave on high for two minutes. Draw cooked egg toward the middle of dish and the liquid egg toward the edges and microwave on high for two minutes more. Sprinkle cheese on top, and microwave until cheese is melted (about 30 seconds more). Let stand a few minutes before serving.

Per serving: 280 calories, 20 g protein, 21 g carbohydrate, 13 g fat, 4.3 g saturated fat, 6.2 g monounsaturated fat, 1.2 g polyunsaturated fat, 218 mg cholesterol, 2.2 g fiber, 296 mg sodium. Calories from fat: 42 percent.

Index

About the Author

Elaine Magee is positively passionate about changing the way America eats—one recipe at a time! Her national column, *The Recipe Doctor*, appears in newspapers such as the *Atlanta Journal-Constitution, Democrat and Chronicle, Hartford Courant, Honolulu Advertiser,* and magazines such as *Today's Health & Wellness.* In the column—which she has been writing for the past decade—she performs recipe "makeovers," in which she is able to bring down the calories, fat, saturated fat, and sometimes sugar and sodium, while at the same time increasing fiber, phytochemicals, omega-3s, and monounsaturated fat. Elaine "doctors" real recipes while retaining the original good taste, and she keeps it easy. She believes that if there is a shortcut in the kitchen, you should take it!

Elaine is the author of more than 25 books on nutrition and healthy cooking, with her most recent book being *Food Synergy* (Rodale, March 2008). Elaine's medical nutrition series includes *Tell Me What to Eat If I Have Diabetes, Tell Me What to Eat If I Have Irritable Bowel Syndrome,* and *Tell Me What to Eat If I Have Acid*

Reflux. Hundreds of thousands of these books have been sold, and they are now being distributed throughout the world, including China, Russia, Spain, Indonesia, and Arab countries. New editions of these three books in the series will be released October–December 2008.

Elaine is a nutrition expert and writer for Webmd.com, SilverPlanet.com, and magazines across the country, and she appears frequently on radio, educational videos, and television shows. She has appeared on *Eye on the Bay* in San Francisco, the Fine Living Network, the *CBS Evening News, Mornings On 2* in San Francisco, and *AM Northwest* in Portland. She also conducted monthly healthy cooking segments for the Saturday morning news on NBC–San Francisco for two years. For two years before that, Elaine performed the "Light Cooking" segment for the KSBW-TV (NBC) midday news in Salinas, California. She was the writer and guest on a video with Teri Garr on multiple sclerosis and with Shekhar Challa, MD, on "The Heartburn Friendly Kitchen."

Elaine graduated as the Nutrition Science Department "Student of the Year" from San Jose State University with a bachelor of science in nutrition and a minor in chemistry. She also obtained her master's degree in public health nutrition from UC-Berkeley and is a registered dietitian. She was a nutrition instructor at Diablo Valley College for two years and the nutrition marketing specialist (California Department of Health) for the now national "5 a Day" health program for three years.

Other recent projects:

- Elaine is getting ready to launch her internet cooking show (stay tuned).
- Elaine was part of a satellite media tour in November 2007 on the topic of heartburn and the holidays.

- Elaine was the recipe developer for Pfizer pharmaceuticals, providing recipes to its Website specific to three medical issues: high blood pressure, high blood cholesterol, and diabetes.

Other Books of Similar Interest

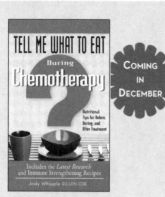

Tell Me What to Eat During Chemotherapy
Nutritional Tips for Before, During, and After Treatment

EAN 978-1-60163-045-2
U.S. $12.99

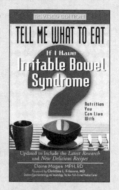

Tell Me What to Eat If I Have Irritable Bowel Syndrome
Nutrition You Can Live With

EAN 978-1-60163-021-6
U.S. $12.99

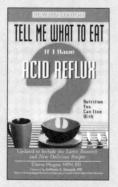

Tell Me What to Eat If I Have Acid Reflux
Nutrition You Can Live With

EAN 978-1-60163-019-3
U.S. $12.99

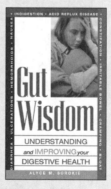

Gut Wisdom
Understanding and Improving Your Digestive Health

EAN 978-1-56414-753-0
U.S. $15.99

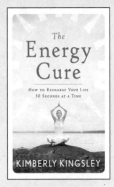
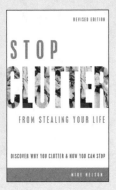
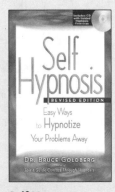
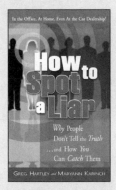